SPIRITUALITY, SEXUALITY AND HIV/AIDS IN MALAWI

Copyright 2006 Augustine Musopole

All rights reserved. No part of this publication may be reproduced, stored in a retrieval system, or transmitted in any form or by any means, electronic, mechanical photocopying, recording or otherwise, without prior permission from the publishers.

Published by
Kachere Series
P.O. Box 1037, Zomba, Malawi

ISBN 99908-81-02-2
Kachere Studies no. 7

The Kachere Series is represented outside Africa by:
African Books Collective Oxford (orders@africanbookscollective.com)
Michigan State University Press East Lansing (msupress@msu.edu)

Layout and Cover Design: Caroline Chihana

Printed by Lightning Source

SPIRITUALITY, SEXUALITY AND HIV/AIDS IN MALAWI

Theological Strategies for Behaviour Change

Augustine Musopole

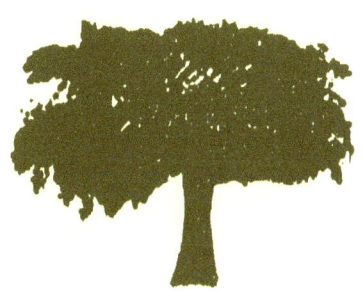

Kachere Studies no. 7
Kachere Series
Zomba
2006

Kachere Series
P.O. Box 1037, Zomba, Malawi
Kachere@globemw.net
www.sdnp.org.mw/kachereserie/

This book is part of the Kachere Series, a range of books on religion, culture and society from Malawi. Related books are:

Frank Ham. *Aids in Africa: how did it ever Happen*

Treasuring the Gift. How to Handle God's Gift of Sex. Sexual Health Learning Activities for Religious Youth Groups

John Dubbey, *Tlamelo. The Church Against Aids*

Klaus Fiedler, *Let's Build the Bridge*

Rachel Nyagondwe Fiedler, *Coming of Age: A Christianized Initiation among Women in Southern Malawi*

Chipo Kanjo, *Will to Live*

Kudzai Nhamo, *A Silent Battle*

Janet Y. Kholowa and Klaus Fiedler, *In the Beginning God Created them Equal*

Masiye Tembo, *Touched by His Grace: A Ngoni Story of Tragedy and Triumph*

Maria Saur, Linda Semu and Stella Hauya Ndau, *A Study of Gender-Based Violence Nkhanza in three Districts of Malawi*

Andy G. Khumbanyiwa, *Better Days Around the Corner. Restoration of Hope, Self Confidence and the Desire to Succeed*

The Kachere Series is the publications arm of the Department of Theology and Religious Studies of the University of Malawi

Series Editors: J. C. Chakanza, Fulata L. Moyo, Chimwemwe Katumbi, F.L. Chingota, Klaus Fiedler, P.A. Kalilombe, Martin Ott, Shareef Mohammad

"Since Aids is a behavioural problem, proposed solutions will not be effective unless they change the behavioural patterns of people."

Fulata Moyo, "The Aids Crisis: A Challenge to the Integrity of the Churches in Malawi" in Kenneth Ross, ed., *Faith at the Frontier of Knowledge*, Blantyre, CLAIM Kachere, 1998.

Preface

It is now twenty years ago since the Executive Committee of the World Council of Churches (WCC) meeting in Reykjavik, Iceland, called upon the churches worldwide to urgently address the issue of Aids. The call arose out of a consultation on the theme, "Aids and the Church as a Healing Community." After twenty years the church in Africa in general and in Malawi in particular is attempting to respond to the crisis that has continued to deepen with devastating consequences for individuals, families, communities and nations, disturbing politics, economy, and the entire social fabric. One reason for the slow response from the churches has been the lack of adequate theological tools and strategies.

The Reykjavik consultation sought to understand the identity of the church as a healing community, a role that is usually associated with medical practitioners only, be they modern or traditional. It is a role that seems not to need theological understanding, only the technical know-how. However, healing is not a matter of taking chemical substances to assuage pain and suffering but rather it is the restoration of life to wholeness. Healing is related to Shalom, peace, which has to do with the restoration of relationships. Therefore, healing is part of the church's responsibility as healing communities. It is not just the body that needs healing, but also the mind, the emotions, the relationships, the spirit. Aids is a disease that affects the whole person and, therefore, there is need for holistic strategies to combat it. The Ryekjavik consultation identified the following theological foundations for the church as a healing community:

1. In the mysteries of life and death we encounter God, this encounter calls forth trust, hope and awe rather than paralysis and immobilization so that those who cannot be cured can be supported and sustained in solidarity in the name of Jesus who is met among the hungry, the sick, the naked, the rejected, the prisoners, and now those living with HIV/Aids (cf. Matt. 25:31 ff)

2. The Aids crisis challenges the church profoundly to be the Church in deed and in truth. It is God's people who are infected and affected by HIV/Aids. Therefore, the church as a healing community needs to be healed by Christ for it to play its role more effectively.

It is this realization that unless the church is clear about the theological foundation for combating HIV/Aids, it's interventions will only remain moralistic and negative to say the least. And yet, the churches in Malawi are weak when it comes to theological reflection, especially in the field of contextual theologies that are needed to relevantly address this matter. The received and inherited theologies that are often mechanically repeated and maintained without much understanding are unable to engage the cultural context in which we live because they were created for a different cultural and historical milieu, and were responding to different questions.

This book is written with a view to providing culturally relevant theological reflection on the issue of Aids and to act as a resource in the combat of Aids especially in bringing about meaningful behaviour change. Unless the churches develop the ability to engage in sustained theological reflection and not simply harp back to denominational tradition that they have received and faithfully maintain even when in their place of origin the churches have moved on and changed with the time, and keep on using proof-texts from the Bible, the efforts to bring about behaviour change will prove futile. This observation that Samuel Terrien made when discussing a biblical theology of manhood and womanhood is also relevant in this current discussion on HIV/Aids. He observed, "When Biblicists of the Roman and sectarian varieties appeal to the 'law of Moses' or the letters of Paul in order to justify obsolete codes of sexual ethics as divinely ordained, their *procedure* [my emphasis] displays a literary fallacy and historical illusion that imply either ignorance or a misapprehension of the way in which biblical literature was written, selected, and slowly 'canonized'". He goes on to remind us that Scripture is an anthology of historical records and then continues to say,

> "Jesus himself proclaimed the need for facing historical change when he observed that new wine required new wine skins. On the other side of the spectrum, contemporary ethicists of sexuality appreciate the meaning of change, but they often ignore the continuity of purpose that permeates the biblical picture of man's and woman's destiny. They risk falling into the transitoriness of moral pragmatism, thus reducing religion to morality and morality to self-interest."[1]

Without proper, adequate and critical theological reflection of the reality of HIV/Aids, the churches in Malawi would also be running the risk of reducing religion to morality, while the secular attempts would run the risk of reducing morality to self interest. Both of these positions would miss the mark to bring about meaningful behaviour change.

---

[1] Samuel Terrien, *Till the Heart Sings*, Philadelphia: Fortress Press, 1985, p. 4.

The theological reflections that follow are meant to stimulate a more comprehensive and deeper reflection on several aspects of this human catastrophy. In order to avoid the dangers described above, the reflection recommends what it calls *Christic realism*. Christic realism is the attitude displayed by Jesus towards similar cases during his time on earth. The critical questions to ask are twofold: What did Jesus do in comparable situations? And, What would Jesus do today?

The reflections attempt to take a step in discussing sexuality without being irresponsible or making it a laughing stock or a joking matter, since it is serious business upon which our future depends. It is an attempt to help the churches to teach faithfully, honestly, and symphathetically instead of usurping God's position as judge. The church is being called to be like the prophet Ezekiel who was told, "Son of man, I am sending you to the Israelites. The people to whom I am sending you are obstinate and stubborn. Say to them, 'This is what the Sovereign LORD says'. And whether they listen or fail to listen—they will know that a prophet has been among them" (Ezekiel 2:3-5). Bringing about behaviour change is fundamentally the work of the Holy Spirit as the Holy Spirit applies God's liberating truth to our lives thereby breaking the power of sin that enslaves us. It is a tough job since it means giving up cherished sources of pleasure. However, the church is called to be there on behalf of a liberating God remaining faithful to the proclamation and teaching of God's liberating word.

These thoughts have been developing over time, but much more so while I was General Secretary of the Malawi Council of Churches (1998-2003). It was during this time that we grappled with bringing out a position statement on condom use. This was followed by a number of national conferences on HIV/Aids sponsored by Norwegian Church Aid when and where I advanced the view that HIV/Aids was a new mission frontier just as David Livingstone decided that the abolition of slavery was his new mission frontier. During my sabbatical at St. Paul's Theological College, Limuru, Kenya (January-May, 2002), I found time to do some research on spirituality and sexuality, the results of which have been incorporated into these reflections. I thank the Principal of St. Paul's Theological College, Professor Godfrey Nguru, for the opportunity of a sabbatical which afforded me the opportunity to develop further these thoughts. My thanks also go to Dorothy, my wife, for editing the initial draft, and to the Kachere editorial team for accepting the manuscript for publication. Last, but not least, my gratitude goes to my late brother Willie Musopole who died in a road accident on 4th February, 2006 for walking with me on this theological journey, especially for having a keen interest in my progress and endeavours. To him I dedicate this book.

Should the reader find things that they disagree with, they are encouraged to contact the writer below so as to be in dialogue with a view to enriching our thinking on this important matter.

Augustine Musopole
Chang Jung Christian University,
Tainan, Taiwan.

Introduction

The devastating effects of HIV/Aids are everywhere. At a visit to any cemetery, be it in rural or urban areas, the number of new graves is telling enough. The increase in the number of orphans and the responsibility for them being taken over by relatives and community social service creates a picture associated with a war zone and yet no guns rang over our nation. The funeral budget has burst expectations and is crippling vital services. The professional sectors are being depleted of the expertise that has taken so long to develop and yet it is wiped out within a short time. Instead of children and grandchildren burying their parents or grandparents, it is the grandparents who are doing it to their children and grand children. There is the heart breaking sorrow of parents burying one child after another and often in quick succession. There is the suffering of the infected and the affected as they care for their loved ones over a long period hoping against hope that somehow they will pull through. This means that they cannot carry out the necessary tasks to sustain themselves. The pastor, minister, priest is kept busy visiting the sick and burying the dead. This is the face of HIV/Aids. It has left its deadly fingers everywhere with its "killer honey".

The above scenario is made worse by a fatalistic attitude in many young people. They simply shrug their shoulders and say, *"Zonse ndi nthawi"* meaning to everything there is a time, quoting the book of Ecclesiastes out of context, or *"Zinalembedwa"* meaning it was so designed by fate and there is little that one could do. There is a carelessness induced by either ignorance or misinformation that thorough washing after sex can prevent infection as I heard some youth sharing this information. While being aware that the honey is poisoned, they still want to keep having it. Sometimes the people do not want to know, believing that ignorance is bliss.

While HIV/Aids is a recent phenomenon, sexual relations on which it loves to ride, are as old as humanity. Even in the wisdom of our cultures, it was recognized that sexual relationships need to be well managed by individuals and society at large. Therefore, sex was surrounded by taboos and other social norms of respect, fear, love and care. It was related to the mystery of life. However, all that hedged it in mystery began to unravel with the coming of independence. It is important that we appreciate this trend in sexual moral decline since 1964 as part of our own undoing to the point that this pandemic has found a way into our very lives.

For the church, HIV/Aids presents a new mission frontier requiring new methods for carrying out its mission of love and compassion. It is not a case of what should we have done to stop this, even though that is relevant, but rather what should be done now that the lion is in the kraal.

It is the aim of this small book to shed some light on the theological dimension of this new mission frontier. This calls for a radical self-examination of our theology and practice of mission. However, the radicalness of the examination should take us back to Jesus' own self-understanding and evangelical practice to see whether we are not where the Pharisees were when Jesus said to them. "Woe to you Pharisees, because you give God a tenth of your mint, rue and all other kinds of garden herbs, but you neglect justice and the love of God. You should have practised the latter without leaving the former undone. Woe to you experts of the law, because you have taken away the key to knowledge. You yourselves have not entered and have hindered those who were entering" (Lk. 11:42, 52).

While the churches are doing a very commendable job in alleviating suffering resulting from HIV/Aids, it is the theological and ethical basis that is supposed to inform this outpouring of service that leaves much to be desired. Therefore, one reason for this publication is to move the debate from its current stalemate and to raise some critical questions to start a process of critical self-examination of our varied Christian heritage in response to the current multi-faceted challenge that is facing us as a church and as a nation. If this publication provokes some reaction on the matter then it will have succeeded in its purpose.

1. Aids and the Missing Theological Factor

It is commonly lamented that the message about Aids has been adequately disseminated throughout the country, but with little corresponding behaviour change. This has led to seeking new ways of packaging the information so that Aids-related communication aims at behaviour change. Missing in this search is a theological dimension that is often forgotten because we think that God is not scientific. However, believing in a God who created the entire universe, nothing could be further from the truth. The church might not be scientific, but God is. The fact that God cannot be quantified or weighed on the scales, or fitted in a test tube, or put under a microscope need not stand in the way of truth. God as a spiritual reality requires spiritual methodologies to be known and faith that is exercised through scientific methodologies is an aspect of the faith that is the entry point into the reality of God. However, since God is a spiritual personal being, faith in God becomes a personal relationship while that in the sciences remains an impersonal relationship.

Theological strategies for Aids prevention and behaviour change must be considered more in the long-term than in the short-term perspective. I consider the condom as more of a short-term crisis management strategy. There is much more at stake in this pandemic than simply prevention of transmission of HIV. Various things are at stake. They include our sense of being human, our understanding of sexuality and its implications for the relationship between men and women, the meaning of our bodies personally and in sexual unions, the psycho-spiritual and social dimensions of sexual intercourse, learning to take responsibility for our sexuality and its appropriate management. It is only in these various contexts that we can meaningfully talk of behaviour change, and theology has much to say about this.

We need to advocate a holistic approach that entails looking at ourselves in the totality of our existential context and not simply as sinners or as preventing disease. HIV/Aids affects the total immune system thereby undermining the capacity of the whole life to function well. Its effects are not only personal, but also communal. Aids impacts on our economic ability and our social networks. In the end, we are all left losers and the poorer for it. The churches can no longer ignore this. They cannot be fighting rearguard battles over condoms, seeking confessions, being vindictive and playing God. They must now go to the frontline and network with all people of good will to seek long-term solutions. The greatest challenge lies in saving the next generation by stopping the spread of HIV/Aids. This calls for raising moral stakes in society through relevant and comprehensive sex education, setting up counselling centres and training people in counselling in anticipation of mental, social, and spiritual problems among so many orphans, who will shortly come of age with impaired ability to cope with life.

Below are some theological strategies to address the problem of behaviour change, which does not appear to be taking place to mitigate the effects of HIV/Aids.

The churches have often seen traditional worldviews and cultures as pagan. This epithet makes them a theological issue and, therefore, integral to the theological strategy. The term pagan, however, does not make theological sense in relation to our traditional ways. It is therefore part of the problem that calls for change of attitude and behaviour. The word pagan comes from Latin and means rural person as opposite to urban dweller. In Malawi we say *anthu akumudzi*. It has nothing to do with being holy or wicked, Christian or non-Christian. However, religious connotations that have been attached to the word are obstacles to dealing with it as a theological phenomenon. Since it is what forms our cultural world, it is the first one that we must deal with.

2. Understanding and Appreciating our Traditional Worldview

Our communication efforts related to HIV/Aids have been limited and misguided. This is because they have ignored African perceptions of sexuality, besides simply condemning certain African cultural practices. The practices that have been condemned are part of a grid of meaning rooted in our people's worldview. A worldview provides the lens through which to make sense of the cosmos and to live in it meaningfully, securely, and harmoniously with all the other realities. Religion underpins this worldview as a system of spiritual relationships maintained by rituals, the power of the word and a variety of activities.

Within the African worldview(s), sexuality is one of those very strong vital forces that make life secure, meaningful and worthwhile. And yet it does not seem to occur to us to analyse reasons why sexually related rituals are found in the practice of agriculture, medicine, business, new establishments including housing, death cleansing rituals, adolescence rites of passage, child growth, travel, religious performances and hunting among others. What is it about sexuality that makes it such a pervasive and potent force?

Sexuality is one of the most profound life forces. It has the secret of life to the point that even the growing of food, the fertility of the land and an abundant harvest depend on sexual rituals. It is so pleasurable that it must be indulged in frequently except when it is prevented by very strong and life threatening taboos. It is an energizing force so that without it people feel dead. It has links with other forces in the cosmos. It links each one of us to past and future generations. By it, our vital relationships with the earth are renewed and, when it is a taboo, then it secures the life of the community from destruction and even death.

The various sexual roles as exercised by men and women in traditional society are deduced from the same worldview. Speaking of the environmental crisis, Jürgen Moltmann states, "the values and convictions which prevail in human societies, and regulate public life, themselves derive from fundamental human convictions about the meaning and purpose of life".[2] This is also true of sexuality in African societies. Such values and roles cannot be changed unless the worldview also changes. Therefore, behaviour is informed by fundamental convictions in a worldview. In order to change behaviour, we need to change the worldview that conditions the mind set and the cultural practices.

Women are considered the passive element. They are a garden that receives the seed. They provide the necessary conditions for growth of the human seed, but they do not contribute to the seed except to provide the necessary nourishment. Like the garden, they are sometimes hot or cold. Barrenness is one of the greatest curses for any one especially and so for a woman. It is considered as death to part of the clan's life and survival. The term barren itself is used more in relationship to land. People do not waste their energy ploughing barren land; they abandon it in search of more productive land. This same attitude is applied to women without child.

The men are considered to be the active element. They have the seed and are the planters. They are supposed to be sexually alive, but from time to time some are found to be sexually dead. Nothing is as humiliating and devastating to manhood as to be found to be impotent. Therefore, the greatest challenge is for men to test their manhood not necessarily with a view to procreation even though that is laudable, but to have an erection, penetrate a woman and deposit the seed in her. With pride they declare that one garden is not enough for a man. The more women they go to bed with, the greater their reputation. They consider themselves as cocks and bulls or he-goats. This imagery, though demeaning, does not prevent the men from behaving sexually at an animal level. It is at this level of thought and activity that HIV/Aids finds the chance to spread. Until men's thinking begins to operate at a higher and nobler level, behaviour will not change.

In the Malawi traditional worldview sexuality and love are concomitant with life and survival. Death diminishes life while birth replenishes it. The proverbial saying, "The calves are the real kraal", denotes that the birth of children is the community's hope for survival. This is one of the reasons why HIV/Aids is such a threat. It is taking away the children leaving behind older people whose strength has waned. Moreover, the link of sexuality to life makes it ritually significant as a power for generating life and renewal.

This is why sexual rituals are so pervasive as to be used in agriculture, business and career promotion and in securing one's life and property. For

---

[2] Jürgen Moltmann, *God in Creation. A New Theology of Creation and the Spirit of God*, New York, 1985, p. 23.

women, sex is used to show appreciation for someone, for saying thank you, for obtaining favours, for securing employment or career promotion and to feel attracted or attached to someone, among others. Female sexuality is also used to manipulate men, whose sexuality is driven by economic and political power. This has reduced sexuality to a matter of function. As long as it can meet the desired ends, it is acceptable regardless of the consequences. The meaning of self is separated from the sexual body parts that are then turned into tools economic or for pleasure ritual.

Traditions in Malawi are ambivalent in their attitude to sexuality. For instance, communities will celebrate the coming of age of girls, but a month later the same girls are surrounded by taboos when they undergo the second menstruation. Similarly, sexuality is a most welcome activity that can also be dangerous. When it takes place within socially accepted norms, it is cause for celebration, but when it takes place outside accepted norms, it is ominous and arouses much anger. In the latter case, something has to be done to repair the breach of communal peace. The man is accused of stirring up trouble for his clan, while the woman is accused of shaming her people, especially her mother and father.

There is need to deal with this gender-based moral ambivalence if we are to promote behaviour change. We need a clear theology for our social norms in relation to sexual development and behaviour of people that will include a theology of the body, of sexuality, and of sexual pleasure and sexual ritual within the context of human inter-relationship in the cosmos.

Our traditions shrouded sexuality in much secrecy. We were told that babies were fished out of water or dug out of an anthill, and more recently that they were bought from the hospital. Initiation ceremonies still occur in remote places and the initiates vow not to divulge what they are taught to those who are yet to be initiated into the mysteries of life. Much of this is about sex education and good behaviour. They still have to learn coded language to identify and distinguish the initiate from the uninitiated ones.

Our people are taught that sexual intercourse should be done in the dark so that they do not see each other's anatomy. This is considered to be part of sexual etiquette since to show off is regarded as the behaviour of prostitutes. In Chitipa, a prostitute is called *umalaya*, meaning the well dressed one. Only prostitutes were unashamedly showy in their dress and make-up. The chiChewa word *hule* is from the English "whore". It followed that self-respecting women would not behave like prostitutes even in their own bedrooms. There had to be little or no discussion except in coded language and with the use of symbolism.

Intimacy was not something for public display because *"masiku sakoma onse"* (not all days are Sundays). It is also said that marriage is an ancient institution so no couple should behave as if they were the first to discover it, therefore, marriage is not something to boast about. As a result, intimate public display of love and sexuality is not encouraged. When Western couples are seen hand in hand, they evoke derisive laughter for their inappropriate behaviour or comments like *"Ichi ndechani"* or *"ichi nchivichi"*, meaning what is this? Other comments are *"Chaza ndi yani?"* meaning, "Where has this behaviour come from?" and *"Hedeee! Uuuiii!"* a ridiculing laughter.

In the light of the above, one begins to understand why Western movies and videos that display that intimacy by graphically revealing the secret mysteries of life, so to speak, offend those who take cultural values seriously. It is tantamount to *kuziyalusa*, meaning to devalue not only the significance of human sexuality, but also to devalue one's humanity and reduce it to an animal level. This goes for radio and TV messages, posters, teaching on condom use and other information devices. This becomes worse when it is the younger informing elders.

Sensitivity to cultural attitudes is critical if there is going to be behaviour change; otherwise, people simply block the message, treat it as unacceptable and continue with their old ways of behaving. For instance, the condom has a lot of implications for adjustment of sexual behaviour. It is not simply about its use, but also the coded message entailed in its advocacy and use by men and women. In the case of married couples, it raises various questions. Why use it? Why accept and encourage unfaithfulness? Who is being unfaithful here? Why should it come between spouses? What about supply of semen for its beneficial properties?

The question of testing raises more questions: What will other people think? What will they say about us? How will they treat us should we test positive? For both men and women, to be involved in all this amounts to *kuziyalusa* (chiChewa), *kujichombola* (chiTumbuka) such that the message generates much fear. Therefore, a critical analysis and appreciation of traditional sexual attitudes by the churches is important if we are to contribute to behaviour change in a meaningful and relevant way.

Modernity has greatly eroded the power of traditional sexual norms. There is today much more public display of sexuality, which is blamed on Western culture. We are now even in the process of enacting policies, which advocate legalization of so-called sex-workers. Sexuality is increasingly becoming a public affair. Many factors that include social mobility, education, communication, videos and TV and globalisation have contributed to the current situation that affects the way men and women behave.

There is confusion as to what constitutes acceptable behaviour even in churches. We are a people in transition on many fronts. We are neither in the past nor are we in the modern period. The bad and the good, the acceptable and the unacceptable are all mixed up in one cultural pot. How do we define and understand the period in which we stand? Who determines what our behaviour is to be as a people and as a nation? How does the Church with its history deal with people living at this point in time? Unless as churches we appreciate the times we are in and learn to apply the word of God relevantly to these times, we cannot contribute to behaviour change in the struggle against the spread of HIV/Aids. Churches have to be theologically assisted in harnessing traditional norms to these modern times, otherwise many of our people are going to live split lives, hear conflicting messages, behave in contradictory ways, and suffer from socio-religious schizophrenia even as they die of Aids.

Our traditional worldview has tended to use negative language when applied to sex and sexuality. The word used for making sexual advances by men, *kunyenga*, in the local language means, "to seduce", "to cheat" "to deceive" with a view to engage in sexual intercourse. The word *chiwerewere* is any illicit sexual relationship including pre- and extra-marital ones. It does not cover legitimate loving marital sexual relationships.

Since Aids is not only spread through sex, the emphasis on *chiwerewere* contributes to shame and stigma for those who may have contracted HIV/Aids within their homes while remaining faithful spouses. They simply got infected through some other means, for instance, through unclean needles and blood transfusions in our health centres in the eighties. The problem is that however contracted, once the virus is in the bloodstream, it is sexually transmitted to innocent partners. And yet, the negative connotations of the word *chiwerewere* attribute to such people a sense of shame. They do not only feel stigmatized, but they are stigmatized and discriminated against.

In our traditional cultures, words for body parts are used to insult others (*kutukwana* in chiChewa and *Kutuka* in chiTumbuka). The worst insults involve private parts of men and women and especially of a mother's sex and excretory organs. The rationality of this negative psychology of put-down and humiliation with regard to what are the most precious and sacred gifts associated with life-giving and nurture is difficult to figure out.

The phenomenon of using body parts to insult and humiliate their owners when we all have them betrays a deep-seated hatred of our bodies, probably fostered by the shame culture or its rejection, therefore demanding freedom to name them publicly. I raise this as a problem in the way of positive behaviour change in sexual attitudes. Is it the uncleanness that is culturally associated with our sexual and alimentary processes that make them be used for the most ugly and humiliating insults? Can it be that engagement in sex is a dirty act? Unless we learn to value other people and respect them as made in God's image, including their sexuality, we cannot expect much change in our behaviour. In chiChewa, there is no word for legitimate sexual union within marriage. We need to find one.

Nothing brings out more laughter, cheers, and jeers than the mention of private organs. When it comes to gender, it is the women's body parts that attract most insults and laughter, cheers and jeers from men. The result is that a cultural attitude of shame has developed around this subject. The only way it can be brought up publicly is in jest. The implications are that the subject of human sexuality can never be taken seriously and discussed publicly as such. It becomes a guessing game between men and women employing hints, coded messages, body language, and takes place under the cover of darkness.

It is important that we look critically at our worldview in order to discover what is humanizing or dehumanizing in it, especially with regard to the whole traditional ideology of sexuality if we are to effect profound behaviour change. We have all, as it were by osmosis, breast-fed from that worldview that informs our behaviour in a very subtle, but profound manner. The problem is that most of the time, we are unaware of this world-

and its underlying philosophical assumptions. We just live it without understanding and appreciating it. For instance, what power do women have in negotiating sex in society? What are the cultural mechanisms for this? How adequate are they? What is it in our culture that makes men think that a woman's 'No' is a prelude to a 'Yes'? Why is a threat to expose someone's sexual advances a greater deterrent than a woman's 'No'? How is the culture of shame making women vulnerable to HIV infection?

Before we blame the culture of shame, fear and respect especially in relation to men that is imposed on women and children and therefore making them vulnerable, we need to consider its positive aspects within the traditional value system in relation to sexual behaviour. Inappropriate sexual behaviour such as incest, rape, child molestation, sexual defilement is common in many cultures and has been criminalized in many cultures. Sex taboos were put in place in order to deter such criminal or inappropriate behaviour. While certain relationships were joking or play relationships (*asewere, kayemba*), others were avoidance relationships (mothers-in-law, fathers-in-law). It is these avoidance relationships that insisted on shame, fear, and respect. Like all good intentions, some cultural norms can be carried to extremes and become oppressive laws in authoritarian situations. It is also true that under unbridled individual freedom certain practices can equally go to extremes. Each culture needs to be guided by its wisdom to decide what is appropriate or inappropriate, when and why. As a stakeholder in any culture, the Church has an important role in this process, which must be entered into democratically as it takes into account both the rights of individuals and those of the community.

3. Understanding God's Culture and Human Sub-Cultures

The traditional Malawian worldview is a subculture established on the creative culture of God. It is God who set the cultural stage on which we discover our own ways of being human in the cosmos. The world is not of our making in spite of the improvements we make on in it. Our Malawian religio-cultural traditions acknowledge the reality of God as *Namalenga, Chauta or Chiuta, Leza* and so on. In this, our religio-cultural traditions and the biblical traditions agree. *Namalenga* is the God of Life. It is a name with a feminine designation pointing to God as creator, nurturer and provider. The religio-cultural traditions' thrust aims at relating harmoniously with all the perceived forces in the universe, promoting good ones and discouraging harmful ones. Our religio-cultural tradition has to do with the maximization of life and the prevention of death. We are hemmed in by these two foci. One of the forces that work for life against death, among other things like food and water, is our sexuality. Sexual taboos are meant to protect life against perceived or unseen dangers since sexuality is closely related to life. The Bible also relates spirituality and sexuality when it states, if I may paraphrase it, "And God made **humanity** in God's own image, in the image of God **humanity** was made, male and female God made **humanity**" (Gen. 1:27)

Both religious traditions emphasise that we are God's creation and uniquely made to relate to God. We speak of the human spirit or human blood as priceless. We also speak of the need to respect humanity. Both traditions value sexuality by acknowledging it throughout one's life: at birth, adolescence, marriage, first birth, menopause, death, and in the spirit world. Therefore, it follows that in both traditions, sexuality cannot be taken lightly without paying a high price personally, socially and in cosmic disturbances.

This being the case, behaviour change relating to sexual activities must cast a wide net to address all the issues especially those affecting the peace of the cosmos and the individual and communal human responsibility in it. Our religio-cultural traditions must be reconciled with the Biblical traditions in order to match the culture of God and our human sub-cultures established on it. This is what cosmic harmony is all about.

4. Understanding Sexuality and its Responsibility

The path of our sexual development is decided upon in the womb. It is our creator God who designed it that way and by creating us after His own image, He also elevated our sexuality and made it different from that of animals. The fact that the image of God gives us a unique relationship with God also gives our sexuality a unique purpose in the plan of God for our lives. It carries an awesome responsibility in the expression of the love of God with those we are sexually in love. More will be said on this later.

A proper understanding of our sexuality and our responsibility for it is very crucial in our search for ways to bring about behaviour change. Sex is a good and terrific gift as Fulata Moyo keeps reminding us through her writings and presentations. It is a very powerful force that calls for a lot of responsibility and discipline in its management. We so easily get addicted to it that marriage had to be created especially for its expression and practice.

Sexual intercourse comes with a zing that leaves one feeling drained. It is more than sweetness; it is the sweetness of life from one to another, a deep sense of being alive. It takes us to the border of life and death, that is, to the very gates of heaven, and back again to earth. It is thus one of the greatest affirmations of abundant life. It creates hope and is, therefore, a promise of more good things to come. It gives us a vision of the fullness of life and a sense of security in a loving relationship. It is this ecstatic pleasure that makes people take risks with each other especially when sexuality remains virtually at the animal, selfish, and self-centred level.

We need to address sexual pleasure and give it theological grounding in order to rescue it and us from animal behaviour. We should see sex as a humanizing activity and the fun that accompanies it as an aspect of the joy of the Spirit and part of the beautiful choreography performed by human beings enjoying the love of God in and through each other. The pleasure is the music accompanying the dance of celebrating love and life. There is nothing to be ashamed of in this. Just as the beauty of each dance is in its varied styles, so it is with the sexual dance when performed for the glory of its maker, God.

What is sexuality? Sexuality is more than sex, which has to do with our biological makeup as male and female and is but a small aspect of sexuality. Sex refers to our sexual apparatus, the genitalia (*kumpheto* in chiChewa, *kumavwalo* in chiTumbuka) and all its paraphernalia. In a man, the penis (*mbolo*) and testicles *(machende)*. The penis is used both as an instrument for draining water from the bladder (*chikhozozo*) and introducing sperms (*mbeu* or *umuna*) into the vagina (*nyini*). However, theologically, with the whole pelvis, it acts as a giving or gifting body part of the self to the other, engaging every other part of the body. The whole life is concentrated here in order to give the whole self to the other. Genitalia are communicative bodies for communion, love and life, joy and pleasure, ecstasy and peace. This is its spiritual and mystical function and contribution. This is why I prefer to call them the sixth sense that is different from touch, sight, sound, smell, and taste. They engage all the other senses in their own expression and activities. In a woman, the apparatus consists of the clitoris also euphemistically called "the bean" and the vagina (*nyini*), a receptacle in which sperms (*mbeu* or *umuna*) are deposited, which extends to the uterus (*chibelekelo*) and fallopian tubes (*kumadzila*). The sexual system extends to the breasts (*mawere*), and rhythmically to the pelvis (*mchiuno*) and through the hormones is wired to the rest of the body. Sexually, women are wired in a significant way that is different from men and this fact needs to be appreciated by both men and women.

Sexuality is what it means to be male and female in a relationship. In Genesis 1:27, sexuality amplifies the meaning of the image of God in accordance with Hebrew poetic parallelism. This is what leads us to conclude that spirituality and sexuality are two sides of the same coin. They have to be thought of as belonging together and to be understood in terms of one another. Therefore, it is not surprising that the imageries of sex and marriage are often used to describe our relationship with God.

Sr. Mary Timothy Prokes in her seminal book, *Towards a Theology of the Body*, defines sexuality as "our human capacity as whole persons to enter into love-giving, life-giving union in and through the body in ways that are appropriate. It is basically the power to share self. Sharing involves giving and receiving and not giving and getting."[3] Since sexuality enables us to be person-gift,

---

[3] Sr. Mary Timothy Prokes, *Towards a Theology of the Body*, Grand Rapids: Eerdmans,

"It is Jesus' revelation concerning divine inner life that gives the context for understanding human sexuality in its fundamental sense as revelatory self-gift. The theology of God's inner life is a 'gift-theology', a faith reflection upon the irrevocable given-ness and receptivity among the divine persons. Faith-based understandings of human sexuality take their starting point in the Trinitarian mystery".[4]

From the above theological understanding, Sr. Prokes sees sexuality as an enduring capacity of the whole person. The call to be person-gift is engraved in our very being from the moment of conception. Sexuality is not encapsulated in our reproductive organs nor is it relegated to the period of life between puberty and the diminishment of genital activity. Rather, the entire body-person is destined for life-giving, love-union and through the body in ways that are appropriate to one's age, one's state of life and commitment. Here is the theology of the body that will enable us to reconnect our sexuality not only to our spirituality, but also to our own God's Trinitarian nature. The Christianity that we have come to embrace in Malawi severed spirituality from various other things, of which sexuality is just one. The result has been our failure to think and act holistically.

In his book, *Becoming Christian: Dimensions of Spiritual Formation*, Bill Leonard states, "Our sexuality is a key factor not only in our relationship with others but also with God. We do not become gender-less in prayer, instead, we bring all that we are, including our sexuality, into that relationship."[5] I wonder how many of us give thanks for sex as we do routinely for food? I also wonder how many of us would pray naked to symbolize what the hymn says, "Just as I am without one plea." We have removed our sexuality far away from God and as a result, the original version of one verse of the hymn *"Tumphatumpha Moyo Wanga"* had to be changed for its sexual connotation in the line *"Mulungu wakwezekatu chio**mbolo** mdziko lako"* to *"Mulungu wakwezekatu chitetezo."* Theologically the sense moved from "redemption" to "security" all because of our sexual concerns as inappropriate in relationship to the worship of God. However, we sing with a lot of force the other hymn, "Rock of Ages" and in it is the line, "Naked come to Thee for dress." What a contradiction! We have a problem at our hands that must be addressed if we are to

---

1996, p. 95.
[4] Ibid., p. 96.
[5] Bill Leonard, *Becoming Christian: Dimensions of Spiritual Formation*, Louisville: Westminster/John Knox Press, 1990, p. 176.

contribute towards behaviour change in Malawi in our effort to fight the spread of HIV/Aids.

Norman Pittenger in his excellent book, *Making Sexuality Human*, writes, "The sexuality of man is the natural and human grounding for his awareness of love in all its beauty and appeal. The point is that human sexuality must be seen in the light of the significance we find in love, and not that love has is to be reduced to the level of 'merely' animal sexuality."[6] He then goes on to say, "Sexual expression is a central and splendid means for bringing love into our relationship, for serving God and serving our fellowmen, and for actualizing in a concrete act the union of our personality with one another."[7]

Let me try to unpack what Pittenger is saying. Firstly, he sees love as something of beauty and appeal. Definitely, if God is love, God can be nothing short of this and so must love. However, that love to find a home, and that home is has our sexuality. Therefore, what makes love important is what tells us how important our sexuality is. It is not our sexuality that tells us what love is. It is, therefore, wrong to refer to sexual intercourse as "making love" as we so often hear in pop songs. Sex does not make love, but love makes sex what it must be, two lives in communion. Secondly, sex gives love a foothold, a ground and a place to be established or to build in our relationship. Thirdly, it becomes a means of serving other people and also serving God, but even much more to know that we are complete only in union with the other person. It is not only a woman who needs a man to feel complete as many men think, but men too are incomplete until they are in a loving union with a woman as "bone of my bones, and flesh of my flesh." We have in our traditions and even within the church a very functional view of sexuality when what we need is a theologically grounded understanding of both love and sex.

Love is the bond that binds together in perfect harmony spirituality and sexuality. We cannot talk of the one without the other; we cannot defile the one without defiling the other and separate them without distorting both. Spirituality and sexuality belong together. The greatest heresy is that they have been treated within the history of Christendom as antithetical to each other. This has had terrible consequences for the faith in that multitudes have been prevented from entering fully into their Christian heritage of abundant life because of it. Once our sexuality is understood in the way we have described it above, then attitudes to it are bound to change because such a

---

[6] Norman Pittenger, *Making Sexuality Human*, Philadelphia: Pilgrim Press, 1970: 42.
[7] Ibid., p. 50.

view calls for much responsibility for both spirituality and sexuality. It is not a choice between the two, but both deserve to be nurtured for God's glory and for our own blessedness. Such an attitudinal change will greatly add to our expressing our sexio-spirituality in appropriate ways and thus reduce transmission of HIV/Aids as people begin to take responsibility for their sexuality and to celebrate it appropriately. This will require much teaching.

We can get some wisdom from Taoism also. Writing on Taoism in "The Jade Dragon", Hsi Lai observes that the West has not yet fully comprehended the intrinsic connection between sexuality and spirituality. He adds, "If sexual activity is to have spiritual significance and if the *ying* and *yang* are to be properly enjoined, then each partner must have the proper attitude and feeling to fully experience the activity. It is for this reason that sexual activity must be undertaken with an attitude of harmony and gentleness."[8] How often does the Church in its marital counselling sessions also emphasise "proper attitude and feeling, harmony and gentleness" or does it simply concentrate on the mechanical side taking care only of their mutual wetness?

It is important to note what His Lai says, "Sexual activity is never to be considered as an end in itself, as it is but part of a larger scheme designed to develop love and the natural exchange of male and female sexual energies. All sexual activity must be embarked on first with mutual respect, love, and great anticipation."[9] It is not only the man that gives, but both exchange life-enhancing elements or blessings. Each gives and receives from the other. Sexuality is a responsible way of being human since it is marked by love. It has a sacred function and must be engaged in appropriate ways if it is to avoid negative repercussions. Failure to use it appropriately for mutual fulfillment leads to unfaithfulness and the result in many cases has been infection with HIV. Appropriate understanding and practice of sexuality can only lead to self-fulfilment and fidelity, and then to the glory of God.

Our sexuality and sexual expression is a human personal and social responsibility. Within African cultural practices and traditions, sexual intercourse is also social intercourse, the uniting of the two families represented in it. To engage in premarital and extra-marital intercourse is to breach the social norms. It is as it were to force a sexio-social relationship on two families that have not formally agreed so to do. It amounts to social rape. When this happens, it becomes criminal behaviour for the man, for

---

[8] His Lai, *The Jade Dragon*, 2000, pp. 13, 102.
[9] Ibid., p. 102.

which he must pay, and shameful behaviour for the woman, for which she must be punished. It is these social elements that are forgotten in the condom debate. Sexual intercourse involves entire communities, not just too people.

There is an urgent need to reconsider the subject of masturbation as an aspect of our being sexual beings. Masturbation could be considered as a response to a cry of the whole being for intimate communion, gifting and being gifted, and celebration of gender relationships when it is socially not possible to do so. The alternatives are prostitution and even rape. It has often been heard from both men and women that when the biological powers for engaging in sexual communion are at their peak one feels as if one could simply grab anyone and anything in order to be fulfilled. For some masturbation is the one way out, others use a prostitute, and a few commit rape. Nature may come to one's aid through what is called wet dreams. However, very often for those with moral qualms it calls for bodily discipline and it is a constant struggle of winning and losing. Domestic rape only points to the almost irresistible power of the force of sexuality. What answer has society for this cry of our being for deeper communion across sexes? Biologically we mature early and yet it takes longer to settle into a marriage and others never settle and yet they remain sexually alive and in need of sexual fulfilment. What ethical options are there for them? More on this subject in the next section.

5. Understanding Sexual Management and Control

It has often been said apologetically, "I couldn't help it. It's nature. One can't control nature." This statement is said more often than not to deny responsibility and to blame it on nature. It is the same old approach that Adam and Eve used. They blamed the snake and eventually God himself. However, that did not prevent them from facing the consequences of their act. It also denies our moral being, which is endowed with a sense of freedom and responsibility and this would imply that we place ourselves at the same level as animals that are driven by instinct. And yet, many of us would not accept this conclusion even though we lack the courage to face our own failure and mistakes, betrayal of trust, and loss of reputation. We would protest against being called 'dog' or 'pig' to the extent of suing for defamation. We might share certain characteristics with animals, but we do not belong to the animal kingdom, rather to a class of our own, the human class or realm. We need to revise our biological classification of living things. It is because we are human beings that love and forgiveness are available to us and are able to restore us to our human state from which we constantly fall. We need not remain captive to evil nature and inclination. Our sexuality and spirituality can be managed and need to be managed.

Sexual energy is a gift of God, the sixth sense, as we have called it. A measure of control is applicable to all the senses even though they are all natural. While they may not be learnt senses or abilities, yet we can learn how to control them. St. Paul tells us, "No temptation has overtaken you that is not common to humanity, God is faithful and will not let you be tempted beyond your power to endure, and with every temptation will also provide a way of escape that you be able to endure it." (1Cor.10.13) There is nothing strange about our sexuality that is specific to any one of us. It is a common gift, variations on a common theme notwithstanding. We can depend on the faithfulness of God the giver of the gift. God has not given us something to harm us, but rather to promote our wellbeing.

Granted that under our freedom as creatures, temptation will often assail us, however, it is not the will of God to allow us to be tempted beyond our capacity. In addition to all this, God provides a way of escape from every temptation and it is important that we look for it and use it. Our failure is our responsibility and cannot be blamed on nature or God for having created such a wonderful gift. It is for not taking God's love and purpose seriously that it becomes a source of temptation. God did not include it in our creation to be a trap, but rather we trap ourselves in its wrong use due to wrong understanding. We need to take responsibility for the misuse and abuse of our sexuality and avoid it at all cost.

Jesus talked of "this wicked and perverse generation." Ours is a generation that seeks sexual gratification as if it were living water in a secular globalising culture that has greatly undermined traditional values and means of sexual management. In order to manage our sexuality in a responsible way befitting our humanity in this kind of world, we need:

- To understand and appreciate what sexuality is in the light of our humanity. However, many of us are exposed to scanty information on this matter and most of what is available is inadequate and distorted and serves our male ideologies rather than our lives. The theology of human sexuality, of the body and of sexual pleasure is lacking. This calls for starting sex education early in life.

- The Church has to teach the youth about sexuality in a comprehensive manner. It has to start in Sunday school. Sex education should not wait until the youth reach puberty. There has to be an intentional initiation at puberty into adulthood. This has to continue for those getting married and for those already married for the enrichment of their married love and sexual life.

- Churches should initiate during the long school holiday camps lasting two weeks for initiation ceremonies for all young people who are attaining the age of 14 in a specific year. The camps have to be separate for boys and girls. This is an attempt to save the next generation through knowledge and moral truth.

- The Church needs to bridge the gap between spirituality and sexuality so that they are seen as two sides of the same coin. Spirituality and sexuality have to be understood in terms of each other. This means and implies that sexuality has spiritual dimensions and spirituality can express itself also in sexual ways.

- Love has to be taught as the source of both spirituality and sexuality because it is the very nature of God, the Creator, in whose image humanity is made. Even though love is the greatest commandment, it has not received the theological attention and reflection that it deserves as the primary theological norm. Therefore, love needs to be taught comprehensively. Love is not simply a sentiment, but the very foundation of life and knowledge. To love is to know and to know is to do and to do is to live in blessedness.

- Sexual intercourse in the context of a permanent loving relationship has sacramental qualities and dimensions. It is not simply bodily desires, but a longing of our being for mutual self-offering in a loving relationship to the other with whom we want to enter into and experience mutual spiritual communion and communication of mutual self-knowledge and appreciation as gifts to each other in mutual sharing of lives. This being the case, sexual intercourse is a matter of transparency, accountability and responsibility. It should be done in the light and not in darkness, traditional norms and practices notwithstanding, in the name of truth and not of deception, in honour and not in dishonour, willingly and not by force. There is nothing to be ashamed of about each other's bodies and responsive actions and reactions. There is nothing to hide from one another and from God who judges the motives of the heart. As we have already said, it brings blessings not only to the two people involved, but to the families, communities, and the world.

- Both men and women have to be active participants in and initiators of sexual activity. This will deepen the relationship and satisfy a life sustaining desire. They will be experimenting in search of the best ways of doing it with bodies that are versatile for that function, and in exploring its meaning and mystery. To be passive as some cultures and men demand of women does not equate to being respectful to men and does not signify faithfulness on women's part. It simply robs both men and women of their God-given and designed fulfilment and heritage.

- Sexual expression is both public and private. Some cultures emphasise public expression while others insist on private expression. Both attitudes have their merits and demerits. In Malawi we insist more on the private. When we walk, we rarely walk side by side and even when we do, women struggle to catch up with male strides. However, the question of how much public display should human sexuality have is an issue that needs to be discussed. It is an issue that confronts us through TV, magazines, fashion, advertising, beauty contests, dance halls, offices, and holiday resorts that have become conference centres. Is it possible to provide some guidelines that people could use to judge different situations for themselves? Do we need to protect the public with censorship? What do we understand by adult viewing? What about the many adults suffering from arrested growth who will behave as teenagers? These are important questions to provide much food for thought. Nevertheless, we need to understand the legal framework as well as the cultural parameters of these spaces.

- There are exercises in which both men and women can practise to develop control systems. The Chinese believe that lack of sexual discipline can cause harm to both sexes. We too in our culture have such beliefs, but they are not clearly articulated. These exercises need to be mutual because both stand to benefit as they increase mutual understanding and trust. Men need to pay more attention to this. Frequent ejaculation can only harm the body and reduce one's chances of a long life according to Chinese wisdom. Have you ever wondered why, on the average, women live much longer than men and yet women work harder and longer in addition to bearing children and giving nurture to all in the family? There is need to develop exercises for the conversion of sexual energy into life-creative energy as part of a spiritual and economic discipline. There may be something to learn from those who have chosen a life of celibacy. How do they manage their sexuality-in-spirituality and vice versa?

- Masturbation has been condemned as sinful, but the theological reasons for this condemnation are not clear. Masturbation is a most prevalent sexual activity. What Onan did comes in no way near masturbation. What Jesus said about lusting in one's heart as amounting to committing adultery, needs to be put in its proper biblical and theological context of divorce. All men are guilty of looking at a woman in admiration, but they also know that masturbation may at times involve mental images of some woman.

Now with delayed marriage due to education and pursuit of careers people either engage in pre-marital sexual relations or resort to masturbation or both. Can the Church legislate on this, or is it better left as a private affair between people, their bodies and their God? We all live by the grace of God in need of constant forgiveness. Each failure is a new failure that deserves to be forgiven upon repentance, yes, up to seven times seventy times. This is grace at work. In order to avoid the accusation of providing an easy view of sin, St. Paul asked a very pertinent question, "Shall we go on sinning so that grace may increase? By no means! We died to sin; how can we live in it any longer?" (Rom. 6:1,2). What is the theological and biblical basis for our codes of discipline within the church? Without the grace of God, who can dare say that they are people without sin? We all need the mercy and forgiveness of God. The church is indeed not a hotel for saints at a party, but a hospital for recovering sinners.

A view may be advanced that masturbation is a cry of the whole being for intimacy, giftedness and celebration of gender relationship. It is a cry that God understands and is able to deal with. In traditional practice, they married early and allowed polygamous marriages as a way of dealing with some of the sexual problems. Today a lot prevents people from getting married early and some do not get married at all. Added to this are the many young widows due to HIV/Aids; how do they deal with their sexuality? Married people with daily access to sex have no moral right to condemn those who have no access to sex and yet their sexual urges are strong, if not even stronger. It could even be argued that there are more sinful sexual relationships even in a marriage, for instance, sexual abuse and domestic violence, sexual denial and embargo just to mention a few.

Is it possible to place masturbation at the same level as the problem of meat offered to idols in the Corinthian church? (See 1 Corinthians 8:1-13) If possible, doing and abstaining can be glorifying to God since all give thanks for their various positions. This is suggested as more food for thought.

6. Understanding Sin, Sexuality, and Human Depravity

I vividly recall in the first year of my secondary schooling a teacher telling us that sexual intercourse was the cause of human failure in the Garden of Eden. The woman was the garden and she possessed the tree in the middle of the garden, the forbidden fruit. Since then, I have heard this interpretation as part of folk theology. This is just a fascinating, but imaginary amplification of what the Genesis story is about. Others have seen the snake as a phallic symbol of male sexuality making advances to the woman. However, a careful reading of the story tells us nothing about sex, thought some about nakedness, and it is this theme that is carried on in chapter three. Wherever nakedness is used in the Bible it is mostly in the context of judgement and it points to utter humiliation and condemnation. Only in chapter one is nakedness used in a positive way by saying, "They were both naked but not ashamed."

The fall or human failure was occasioned by the serpent (and whatever it represented) who contradicted the Word of God and turned it into a lie. The serpent further presented an alternative view of what life could be like. Therefore Eve was tempted into disobedience while knowing well what they had been told. What is most surprising though is that Adam is present but silent. He only receives the fruit at the end of the conversation and he too eats it. The catch in the temptation was the denial of death as a consequence and a prospect of being like God. This amounted to denying their 'creaturehood' (i.e. their nature as creatures) and desiring to become like God. It was a temptation to absolute freedom in the same way that God is free. Indeed their eyes got open, but only to realise that they were naked. Their glory was gone and they had to find an immediate solution.

Sin is real, but the nature, power, and consequences of sin are often not well appreciated. The result is that we are being constantly messed up by it and are messing ourselves up in it. Sin is a negative life force, a parasitic spiritual reality, feeding on the good of God's creation and thriving on it. Sexuality is one area where it loves to feed itself. Sin is a power of death and not life, of hatred and not love, of ignorance and not knowledge, of foolishness and not wisdom, of wickedness and not righteousness, of injustice and not justice, of a curse and not a blessing, a source of decay and not growth. It is a spiritual force and coming out of this power are acts of sin that manifest themselves as symptoms of the presence of the Power of Sin. The consequences of sin are corruption, moral decay, and death. Jesus referred to this when he said, "the thief only comes to steal, kill and destroy." And he juxtaposed this with his own mission: "I have come that they may have life and life in all its fullness" (John 10:10)

All of us are aware of sin and that we are sinners, that is, under the power of sin, and as a result we keep on falling short of our true humanity as seen in Christ. (Rom. 3:23) What St. Paul describes below is a common experience of our contradictory sinful lives: "I do not understand what I do. For what I want to do I do not do, but what I hate I do. And if I do what I do not want to do, I agree that the law is good. As it is, it is no longer I myself that it, but it is sin living in me. I know that nothing good lives in me, that is my sinful nature. For I have the desire to do what is good, but I cannot carry it out. For what I do is not the good that I want to do; no, the evil I do not want to do – this I keep on doing. Now if I do what I do not want to do, it is no longer I who it, but it is sin living in me that does it." (Rom. 7:15-20) Sin turns us into walking and breathing human contradictions. This is what human depravity means, that is, living at the subhuman level. This level of existence affects our thoughts and attitudes to spirituality and sexuality leading to idolatry and animal behaviour respectively.

Sin is not only personal, but also societal and structural. It impacts on the entire society and all it's structures. It is national, global, as well as cosmic in its dimensions. All nations have their favourite sins or propensity towards them. Ideologies are equally prone to sin and can be sinful.

Sin, as a human pathology, is historical. It grows, spreads, mutates, and multiplies. It induces moral paralysis and decay in individuals, families, communities, nations, and globally. It takes on the spirit of each culture.

Sin removes us from our God-given humanity to a subhuman level of existence. This is an abnormal level of being human. Since we are born within such abnormal cultures and grow up in them, it seems to us that being sinners is the normal way of being human while it is not. Being so used to evil, we do not find anything really wrong. All our civilisation and progress operate at this sin-oriented sub-human level. As long as the new humanity as seen in the face of Christ is not acknowledged as the life that enlightens every person in all cultures, this subhuman culture is bound to persist in spite of our technological advances. It is only in Jesus Christ that we can be set free from this infection and be put on the path to recovery. We are born again to a new way of being human, Christ's way.

The Bible defines sin in a variety of ways. One such definition is that sin is the missing of the mark; at least that is what the Greek word for sin means. What mark is this, if not the mark of our authentic humanity as created in the image of God, an image shattered by sin, but restored in Jesus Christ? Sin is the failure to obtain the authentic *uMunthu* (humanness).

The Bible also defines sin as lawlessness, but which law if not the law of living our humanity fully and responsibly? Sin is the autonomy we claim only to end up as beasts with a human face because of sin. We are never the gods we thought we might become.

The Bible states that we have all sinned and fall short of the glory of God, but which glory if not the glory of our authentic humanity as created in the beginning and restored in Jesus Christ, the Son of the Human One?

This total failure to have authentic humanness manifests itself in and affects human sexuality and spirituality in a variety of ways. The following are some of the ways:

- Distorted and irresponsible view of love, sexuality and the body
- A distorted view of manhood as centred around the genitalia
- The treatment of women as sex objects, prostitution, and rape
- The commercialization of women's sexuality through prostitution, sex favours, and pornographic literature and films
- Passivity in the socialisation of the girl child
- Cultural rituals and sexual practices that are not moral and various other normal
- Sexual violence, violation, defilement, incest forms of wickedness and injustices related to sexual practices
- Hypocrisy in the church and the failure of the church not only to denounce sin and evil, but to insist on a spirituality without sexuality, and a sexuality without spirituality in its teaching over two millennia.

These are symptoms of the real problem of the power of sin in our lives. All of us know that symptoms point to a disease and that they do not cause the disease and, therefore, we do not treat symptoms in order to deal with the disease. Unfortunately, the churches have been treating symptoms in order to address the problem of the Power of Sin and as a result, the disease (be it sin itself or Aids) has been spreading and becoming more infectious. We cannot ignore to address the issue of the Power of Sin and Acts of Sin in relation to HIV/Aids as a general human condition whether infected or not infected. However, while we cannot impute sin to every sufferer of HIV/Aids, we can expect God to show forth his glory in the sufferer.

The human crisis of HIV/Aids is much greater and deeper than the matter of sexual immorality and condoms. We need to get to the bottom of this problem in our attempts to find lasting behaviour change solutions. Therefore, understanding and appreciating the nature and character of Satan, sin, temptation, and how God deals with all these in grace and forgiveness, will greatly contribute to lessening guilt, fear of hell, stigma and discrimination. It will also bring about peace of mind, love, faith and hope in the way that the future is faced.

This symptom approach to sin has overvalued the sexual sins in terms of their gravity and yet there is no biblical warrant for this attitude. In the Chitipa and Karonga districts of Malawi, the genital area is referred to as *Kumbibi,* meaning the place of sin, while the Bible says it is the heart, that is deceitful and extremely corrupt. (Jer. 17:9) In the story of the woman caught in adultery, one of the things that Jesus' attitude and action teaches us is that sin should not be so over-valued, but rather the redemption of the person and especially so when the accusers are equally guilty. Among the things that Jesus mentions as defiling to the body is foolishness in the same vein as adultery and fornication. There is no theological justification for making sexual sins deserving of greater condemnation than foolishness. Foolishness and adultery are all Acts of Sin that are symptoms of the Power of Sin needing God's mercy and forgiveness. It is hypocrisy and injustice to condemn one and ignore the other. If we are going to ignore the sin of one, we might as well ignore the sins of all in the name of justice and fairness. The proper valuation of sexual sins in relation to other sins should undermine attitudes of judgement, condemnation, discrimination and stigma towards those that are infected and affected.

The answer to this problem of the Power of Sin is what Jesus told Nicodemus, "You must be born again of water and the Spirit." And John also confirmed this message when he wrote, "No one who is born of God will continue to sin, because God's seed remains in him, he cannot go on sinning because he has been born of God." (1 John 3:9 NIV). This is God's grand way of escape from the grip of the Power of Sin. This way of redemption redeems also our wrong sinful attitudes about sexuality and spirituality. Such a solution can only come with relevant and comprehensive teaching about the new humanity. Faith in Jesus through the agency of the

Holy Spirit breaks the Power of Sin over our lives and stops the habitual behaviour of sinning and instead we begin to learn the habits of righteousness. Acts of Sin become accidental traps in which we get caught, but are rescued by the Good Shepherd.

7. Understanding Love and Sexuality

The secular world has brought much confusion in its understanding of love and sex by conflating the two as synonyms. It refers to having sex as "making love" and so even animals make love. Nothing could be farther from the truth. While love may lead to sexual intercourse some of the time, sexual intercourse as such does not generate love. Meaningful sexual relationships begin with "real love" and not infatuation. With real love, sexual intercourse becomes the icing on the cake. The violence often related to sexual matters makes it very clear that in such a relationship love was not even there in the first place. Furthermore, love is much greater than simply genital coupling.

Love is one, but expresses itself in a variety of ways. One way in which love expresses itself is through our sexuality. Not every loving relationship is sexual just as not every sexual relationship is love. However, whenever love and sexuality exist, they can bring the greatest good to humanity since they are both rooted in God.

Let me make reference again to Norman Pittenger's book. He states,

> "No theology, and no religion that fails to put God as love in the very center of its thinking can claim to be Christian. Since love is the meaning of the whole Christian enterprise our failure to make this obvious to the whole world is more than an omission: It is a denial of all that Christianity stands for and means, not only in respect to men, but also in respect to God's nature and his way of acting in the world."[10]

Meaningful and fulfilling sexuality is rooted in God. Pittenger laments the prevalent attitude that treats sexuality as less spiritual, or even as not spiritual at all. He says, "Sometimes, indeed, the attitude has been one of regret for man's sexual drive – it is accepted as a fact, but regarded as a rather unhappy and unfortunate fact." =(Ibid. p.9) We are not animals when we are celebrating two of God's great gifts, namely love and sexuality.

In his book, *The Ethics of Sex* (1964), Helmut Thielicke makes the same observation. "If the bios of man is also not simply identical with the bios of

---

[10] Norman Pittenger, *Making Sexuality Human*, p. 92.

the animals, then sexuality of man, despite parallelism in physiological processes, is also not simply identical with the sexuality of the animals."[11] Our being human elevates our sexuality beyond the animal instinct, just as it elevates our appetite beyond the animal appetite. Our gratitude turns our sexuality and our appetites into means of acknowledging and worshipping God. Therefore, how do we describe this intimate relationship between love and sexuality?

Love recognises the human value beyond "animality" or animalhood and mere function. Thielicke again states, "to regard man merely as the bearer of a function, a functionary, is to dehumanize and make a thing of him, and therefore to enslave him or her. Therefore, the being and function of man are coordinated in some more profound ways. It is in human sexuality that these two converge. More precisely, it is in the choice of the erotic partner, where the personal element is extremely different in different cases."[12] In our sinfulness we generate a very functional view of our sexual relationships due to an inadequate understanding of love and a self-centred existence that aims at using others and not serving them.

In chiChewa, the word for love is *chikondi* and its verb is *kukonda*. It is also used when referring to some place, somewhere one feels at home, comfortable, well settled, and having a sense of being blessed. The same verb in chiTumbuka and other languages, for instance, chiLambya and chiNdali, means to be saturated with something, or to be actually fed up. It is to have too much of something and to loathe it. In some Bantu languages, for instance, Kinyarwanda, the word for love is *kugunda* and yet in Tumbuka such a word has sexual intercourse connotations. However, *kugunda* in chiChewa means to knock as when cattle are fighting. With a little imagination, it might not be knocking with heads, but rather with the pelvic area. Therefore, love and sexual intercourse are not far apart in the thinking of Bantu peoples among whom the Chewa and Tumbuka belong.

While chiChewa has nouns for adultery (*chigololo*) and fornication (*chiwerewere*), the language has no noun for legitimate sexual intercourse. It is described and not named. Even when described, it feels as if one is cursing someone or undressing someone. Therefore, silence is preferred to describing it. I am taking a great cultural risk here. "How can someone undress us in a book like that?" I can hear. Unfortunately, it is the HIV/Aids pandemic that is making us to undress ourselves.

---

[11] Helmut Thielicke, *The Ethics of Sex*, Grand Rapids: Baker Book House, 1964, p. 20.
[12] Ibid., p. 21.

In chiChewa the verb *"kukwata"* means to have sex. It is used for men doing it and not women. For women it is the passive form that is used. The *kukwata* is done to them. From this word come the nouns, *chikwati* or *ukwati* and the verbs *kukwatira* and *kukwatiwa*. In the chiNdali language, the verb *kukwata* means to wear. As the sword is to the sheaf, so is the sheaf to the sword. It is used of clothes that one slips on. It carries connotations of entering into something or covering oneself with something. Because of the mutuality of the experience, other words are used like *kukwatana* or *kugonana* meaning to mutually engage actively in the sexual act. This expression stretches the meaning of sleeping a bit and brings in the woman as an active participant. The words are descriptions and not names of the sexual activity. It seems to me that the verb *kukwata* points to morally acceptable and legitimate sexual relationships since it gave rise to the nouns *chikwati* and *ukwati* for legitimate and acceptable relationships. Unfortunately, with the advent of Christianity, this sense has been complicated by what is called *ukwati woyera* and *ukwati wachikunja*, meaning a holy and a pagan wedding. It is the former that is now being regarded as legitimate while the latter is illegitimate. The critical question is what makes a marriage legitimate and blessed? As churches we may need to revisit our teaching on marriage in view of our African practices and current challenges. Doctrines are located in time and in cultures even though they might be rooted in Scriptures and traditions. However, a clarification of all these questions would go a long way towards helping our people make informed decisions in relation to behaviour change.

The Greeks had four words to express different kinds of love and affection. They had *philia* for friendship, *storge* for family love, *eros* for sexual love, and *agape* for selfless love. Agape, according to the New Testament commentator, William Barclay, is the invincible good will for the beloved. It is the love that prays for the enemy and proceeds to do them what is good. It is out of this understanding that Jesus taught his disciples, "I tell you, love your enemies and pray for those who persecute you." (Matt. 5:44) and St. Paul reminds the Christians in Rome, "If your enemy is hungry, feed him; if he is thirsty, give him something to drink. In doing this, you will heap burning coals on his head. Do not be overcome by evil, but overcome evil with good." (Rom. 12:19-21)

Thus Thielicke states "*Agape* is not a response to a 'love-worthiness' which is already there; rather the creative cause that produces the 'love-worthiness."[13] Speaking of its source, he says, "Agape is not at the man's disposal; nor is it like *eros*, inherent in his nature. Only God can bestow it upon him. Man can be empowered to possess *agape*."[14] This is the love that the world is longing for and yet does not know where to get it. It belongs to the nature of God, who is its only source. It is actually poured into our hearts by the Holy Spirit. (Rom. 5:5) It is *agape* which constitutes our worthiness because it loves me in spite of myself. It takes care of my negative qualities with a view to redeeming them and substituting them with its own beauty.

The implication of adopting *agape* in our sexuality is that again, according to Thielicke, "*Agape* makes neighbour of the sex partner. It recognises their eternal destiny in God. In *agape* I no longer identify the other person with the opposition in which he/she stands to me; nor do I identify him/her with his/her functions, which are directed upon me. I see in him/her as the child of God, and therefore, a dimension that transcends this function."[15] This is the very opposite of what our cultural love teaches us with its biased orientation towards the self and all that the self is related to: my own relatives, my own village, my own tribe, my own region etc. Such cultural love is very functional. It fails to go beyond a utilitarian vision and as such turns other people into tools to be used, men and women turning each other into instruments for personal gain and competition. Agape reaches to my humanity and sees the image of God though faintly and cleanses it so that its true radiance can be seen even afar. Agape delights not only in humanizing the other, but also in serving them. To that effect Jesus said, "Greater love has no one than this, that he lay down his life for his friends." (Jn. 15:13)

Sexual intercourse is awesome business that has a personal character and responsibility and, therefore, agape has to have a central role in it. Having been created in the image of God, it means we have the capacity to exercise agape once we have been redeemed from our subhuman state of and in sin. There is need to respect the eternal destiny, which is conditioned by God in the other. To make their being a means to an end, a mere bridge, a mere instrument of sexual ecstasy, is equivalent to their becoming merely tools, that is, turning them into a thing, an object and not a subject. Thielicke observes, "The person to whom I relate erotically must be my neighbour and hence the object of *agape*. Otherwise, I dehumanize them."[16] He continues:

---

[13] Ibid., p. 32.
[14] Ibid., p. 33.
[15] Ibid., p. 32.
[16] Ibid., p. 34.

"The sex impulse is the desire, accompanied by pleasure and the urge to consummate this pleasure in ecstasy, for psycho–spiritual and physical union with another human being of the opposite sex."[17] He agrees with Nietzsche who said, "all pleasure, all joy wants eternity, wants deep eternity" and then goes on, "in sexual intercourse we are in search of deep, deep eternity." These sentiments can make sense only when agape is known in and through the love that God has for us. John states, "This is love: not that we loved God, but that he loved us and sent his Son as an atoning sacrifice for our sins." (4:10). It is this perspective on our sexuality that carries with it the implication that "Where sexual union is only for animal pleasure without the personal element it turns into aversion, repulsion, disgust upon completion. The personal character of intercourse which includes gratitude and fulfillment are absent, however, it is these that survive the moment of orgasm. It is moments of gratitude that are only expressions, culminations, and concentrations of a continuing relationship which outlasts all changes of mood and feeling."[18]

Many in Malawi are victims of a Christianity that has split spirit from body and are troubled by sexual feelings. I am of the opinion that traditional views of sexuality are in many ways healthier than Christian views. In the traditional view, the spirituality of the sexual relationship is tied to its function. However, the Christian dualistic attitude can be overcome only when we combine the two. To this end Helmut Thielicke remarks, "But if the body is regarded as a mode of being-one's-self and not merely an inferior part of this being-one's-self, then one may also regard the physical *libido* as a mode of this being-one's-self and not merely a possible demonic antagonism of this self."[19] What is he driving at?

Firstly, the word *libido* means the raw sexual energy or feeling with all the accompanying longing for sexual pleasure. In chiChewa it is called *nyele*. It is that pleasurable itch usually spread out throughout the body and it drives us sexually towards someone of the opposite sex. It often develops into a force that cannot be ignored as it seeks to grasp one's total attention until it has been attended to or distracted by something greater. It becomes the excuse that many use when they say, "Nature cannot be controlled." It is there from childhood, but blossoms during adolescence and continues to be a strong current of pleasurable feelings.

---

[17] Ibid., p. 35.
[18] Ibid., p. 38.
[19] Ibid., p. 45.

Secondly, Thielicke is saying that there is nothing demonic about this bodily feeling. It is part of who we are as made in the image of God. The critical question that we need to ask is what does *libido* contribute to the total meaning of being human and the enjoyment of the fullness of life? There is a depth of meaning to our *nyele* and we need to discover that meaning.

Thielicke continues. "There is something in the structure of the *libido* itself that points to a two-way communication, in any case to the rudiments of such possibility; for the prerequisite for the fulfillment of the pleasure is that the other person gives themselves to it, that they participate. But this giving of oneself cannot mean that he/she merely puts himself/herself 'at the disposal' of the other person merely as an object to perform certain functions. Rather it implies that he/she must feel that he/she is 'carried along', and doing so spontaneously, that is to say, on the basis of his/her own *libido*."[20] This goes against the cultural advice of sexual passivity given to women and against the male attitude of viewing women only as instruments. It calls for mutually active participation, recognition of differences in our sexual drives, and the need for mutual care and togetherness. This difference in our sexual responses between men and women is part of God's design for good sexual relationships. It is like two people dancing to the music they love and enjoy. Each responds to it differently, yet they are able to synchronise their dance movements to create something beautiful for their mutual delight and celebration of the fullness of life at that moment in time.

Thielicke is very much concerned that men should take their sexual responsibilities seriously by paying attention with agape to the sexual needs and satisfaction of both and not simply their own. This failure may be at the root of promiscuous behaviour that is helping to spread HIV. Therefore addressing this matter from a theological perspective may contribute to the defence against the virus. Furthermore, Thielicke observes, "The difference between the sexual nature of man and woman does not allow human beings merely to follow the impulse in blind animal fashion, if the urge is to be satisfied. This difference, theologically, confronts us with a task, which challenges us to transcend the purely natural. The creatureliness of the human body is something more and something different from its naturalness. Creaturehood implies that man is challenged at every moment to transcend nature though associated and related to nature. The body along with its *libido*

---

[20] Ibid., p. 46.

is representative of the man himself... it confronts him/her with the theme of human communication instead of merely animal copulation."[21]

Human beings belong theologically to a class of their own. They cannot be compared to dogs, cats, cocks, he-goat, bulls and snakes, as is very often the case. We engage in dehumanising language to our own peril and at great cost to our girl-child and a deformation of the male mindset. Now it is the pandemic that we are reaping from our dehumanising language of male licentious behaviour. Therefore, change of behaviour means change of our language and sexual attitudes, and beginning to celebrate our sexual differences and not making them causes for fighting and dominion.

Being people endowed with reason, a sense of wisdom, and being different from animals, we learn to control nature in many things. We cut our nails and hair when they become too long, we dig and build pit-latrines so that we do not evacuate our bowels the way animals do in the open without any sense of shame. Therefore, we need not become slaves of libido no matter how powerful and pleasurable it may be. It is in this light that Thielicke describes the real function and nature of *libido* when he says, "The human libido cannot just desire only itself, when it desires itself, it must take the other person into account. It must affirm the other person and it cannot only desire him/her. The *libido* must have in it a 'diaconic' element, an element of serving love, if it is not to be left by itself and cheated of its own goal."[22] When we bring a sense of agape to our *libido*, then and only then do we discover the deep meaning of both agape and *libido*.

This explains why rape is a crime and women's mode of dress cannot be used as the excuse. It is our mental attitude that must be blamed. It is a criminal mind that commits rape. Unless men are taught all this as part of their growing up with a view to taking a responsible attitude for their sexuality, behaviour change cannot take place and, therefore, prevention of the spread of HIV/Aids cannot be achieved.

Human beings are not animals controlled by instinct, because as Thielicke continues to enlighten us, "The human sexual instinct demands in the totality of communication to become a motive... For every human sexual encounter becomes a reality only as the partners give themselves to each other, only as one desires to bring sexual joy to the other and thus desires to serve him/her." This is how agape makes its presence felt because it "takes hold of a tendency, which is built into the creaturely sex nature of man in the

---

[21] Ibid., p. 47.
[22] Ibid., p. 48.

form of a sign (for deeper relation) a challenge, and transforms it into a motive. It gives meaning and purpose to what instinct may do ignorantly and relates it to the whole of human existence and community for which man was created."[23] When instinct is linked to the human spirit created in the image of God, it becomes enlightened, morally responsible, theologically meaningful, and trainable. The training of animals is based on their natural instinct that gives them the propensity to achieve new techniques. Therefore, it follows that "where agape permeates the Sex encounter the happiness of the other person is sought in the whole breadth of common existence."[24] The Christian traditions on spirituality and sexuality that Malawi has inherited brought with it a theological worldview that was characterised by a dualistic thinking that has affected Christian practice adversely. The split of nature and the divine, matter and spirit, head and heart, is what is causing problems in our attitude to sex and sexuality. They are treated like tolerated evils.

Much of this attitude can be traced back to the Church Fathers. Making reference to St. Augustine on this issue, Monsignor D. Conway in a foreword to a book by Joseph and Lois Bird states,

> "Catholic teachings about marriage, from the fifth century to the fifteenth century, and even to our own time, were dominated by the doctrine of St. Augustine. For him the love between husband and wife involved too much concupiscence to be sanctifying. Indeed this love could hardly be expressed at all without some measure of sin. Only procreation justified intercourse; so the normal expression of marital love could not be lawful unless procreation were both possible and intended."[25]

This heritage has affected us as well in Malawi. It needs to be put right if we are to develop healthy sexual attitudes that will help us mitigate the effects of HIV/Aids.

We have to strongly reject the temptation of separating spirituality and sexuality, of tearing our soul from our bodies. In support of this rejection, Thielicke writes, "Theologically *libido* and agape cannot be separated. Segregation of higher and lower leads either to indifference to the elemental realm or to its demonization. Both libido and agape are human dimensions which are supposed to work in tandem and not against each other."[26] All this goes against a Christianity that separates *zathupi* and *zauzimu* based on a

---

[23] Ibid., p. 48.
[24] Ibid., p. 49.
[25] Joseph and Lois Bird, *The Freedom of Sexual Love*, St. Paul: 2001, p. 13
[26] Helmut Thielicke, *Sexual Ethics*, Grand Rapids: Baker Book House, p. 49.

distortion of Pauline teaching and a misunderstanding of the implication of the incarnation for our existence. However, even Thielicke is not completely free from this dualistic thinking as seen in his regard of *libido* as the lower element and agape as the higher. They all come from the mind of God.

What follows is the heart of the matter. A split has occurred between the mystery of sexuality and that of humanity, and between these two and the mystery of life itself. We have put asunder what God has put together. This is tragic indeed to say the least. The problem is that it is very easy to pull these realities apart, but difficult to put them together again. Once again Thielicke hits the nail on the head when he states categorically, "the mystery of sexuality reveals itself only when the mystery of humanity and what it is intended to be is revealed and only when love is perceived to be the very theme of life itself."[27] The Birds agree with this view when they write, "It is love which gives sexuality its beauty, which gives it purpose. And it is love which makes it a sanctifying act. While it is a physical act, it is transcended through mutual love and becomes a spiritual experience. If it has to have meaning the two are inseparable."[28] In its Guidelines for Education within the Family, the Pontifical Council for Family Life states, "Human love hence embraces the body, and the body also expresses spiritual love. Therefore, sexuality is not something purely biological, rather it concerns the intimate nucleus of the person."[29]

We have asserted above that sexual intercourse is serious business. Actually it has epistemological significance. It is not only a source of knowledge, but also a method of interpersonal knowledge. Once again, Thielicke describes the quality of this knowledge when he says, "sexual knowledge is qualitatively different from knowledge about sex. It is a kind of knowing from inside. It has to do with self-knowledge in the process of knowing the other. This is the way of love, of sex, of faith." This requires a deep and lasting relationship and should lead to rich and blessed living for all concerned.

The statement continues, "Just as the mystery of the person is enclosed in the husk of sexuality, so his/her person comes to himself/herself only in sexuality and also becomes the object of its self-knowledge. But since on the other hand sexuality points beyond its physical ingredient, this coming to oneself takes place not only in the erotic encounter, but also in the agape

---

[27] Ibid., p. 51.
[28] Joseph and Lois Bird, *The Freedom of Sexual Love*, p. 25.
[29] Pontifical Council for Family Life, *The Truth and Meaning of Human Sexuality*, Nairobi: Paulines Publications, 1997, p. 6.

encounter with other people."[30] Since the physical apparatus of our sexuality conditions many men and women, they often fail to transcend that aspect of our sexuality because they have not known what agape, that invincible good will towards the beloved person, is all about. They are like an engine that lacks the capacity to pull in the higher ranges of our humanity. Agape gives to our *libido* that sacramental meaning and flight that brings heaven on earth and earth to heaven. The separation of the two was a great theological error. Therefore, Thielicke, sees agape as having a deeper perception of human reality when he says "Agape penetrates beyond the superficialities of the momentary adequacies or inadequacies of the other person and addresses itself to their ultimate mystery."[31]

All this information remains mere theory unless it is taught systematically as part of Christian living. It has to be internalised and embodied in a personal philosophy of life if it has to help in the fight against the spread of HIV/Aids by helping people change their attitudes and, therefore, their behaviour. Sexuality cannot be legislated against nor is the fear of hell adequate to stop people from indulging in dangerous illicit sex. Men have to be the primary target. They have to be given the truth because only the truth liberates. Jesus is the embodiment of that truth and he is calling us to embody truth in him and through him if we are to be authentic men, as he is the portrait of authentic humanity. Too many of us live at our biological and animal level having failed to grow into mature human-hood (*uMunthu*), let alone "to the whole measure of the fullness of Christ" (Eph. 4:13)

8. Understanding Sexuality and Theology of *uMunthu*

We are humans and not animals. We are men and women and not cocks and hens. We are human beings made in the image of God. What has all this to do with sexuality? [With everything in and over the world, since we are created in the image of God as sexual beings and called to be stewards in the world.] We need to understand what it means to be a man and a woman as separate and then as man and woman in relation.

The theology of *uMunthu* has to do with the with-us-ness of God, that is, the Divine Reality as Immanuel. According to Scripture, human beings are not only created by God like all the other creatures, but are created in a special and unique way. Human beings are created out of love, with love, in love, through love, by love and for love. They are created for a very unique

---

[30] Ibid., p. 80.
[31] Ibid., p. 98.

relationship with God, with themselves and each other, and also with the environment. They are created with responsibilities. The source of all this is traced to the very life and nature of God. God is LOVE because God is LIFE and God is LIFE because God is LOVE. The life of God is one of love through and through and the love of God is life-creating, life giving, and life-sustaining through and through. God's Life and Love are one and the same. Therefore, where there is love, there is also life, and where there is life-in-God, there is God.

Human beings are made in the image of God as *anthu* and in possession of *uMunthu* as distinct from animals, *nyama*, with *unyama*. To be human is to have the life of love as God has. This loving life is expressed in relations human beings have with God, with themselves, with others, and with their environment or other creatures. Therefore, anything that does not proceed out of love is inhuman, evil, sinful, ungodly, wicked, unjust, and a force for death. It follows that every part of our bodies and lives has to have full love as the power that moves them. As we have already seen, love is the only thing that unites spirituality and sexuality in perfect harmony. It also means that our sense of manhood and womanhood can only be true to our humanity if they are steeped in and formed by love and informed by a theology of love as outline above.

To be human means living and maintaining a character of *uMunthu* in relations. As John Mbiti has expressed it, "I am because we are, and since we are, therefore, I am" becomes the essence of this character and identity. There is a relationship with oneself, with and among others, with one's total environment, and a relationship with God. All these relationships have to be maintained in love. This is an awesome task and a huge undertaking indeed that has to be taken seriously. The roles include personal management, responsible parenthood, resource management, and cosmic priestly function on behalf of all other created things.

To be human means to communicate in love, with love, by love, through love, and for love. When we do not do this it means that we are alienated from our essential *uMunthu*, from one another, from a loving and peaceful social environment and from God who is full of love and compassion. Therefore, if we are true to our humanity and humanness, care and compassion is needed, and should come much before and not after HIV/Aids has infected someone else or when they are no more. This means the care of each other bodies as well. What does it profit a man to win all the women in the world and then lose not only his own life, but theirs as well? What will it profit a woman to win all the men in the world and then lose not only her own life, but theirs as well? However, in the case of HIV/Aids, it is not only losing one's own life, but also putting the lives of many more in jeopardy for generations to come. Whole communities are being decimated for lack of initial loving concern and care.

To have *uMunthu* means to have moral integrity coupled with responsible economic living. It is to refuse to survive on the blood and sweat of other people. Sexuality cannot be used for economic survival. To be either a buyer or seller of sex is to lack moral integrity and a responsible attitude towards legitimate economic productivity. There is nothing more inhuman than to commodify and commercialize part of our bodies. It is worse than slavery since we are willing sellers and willing buyers. Women devalue themselves to sex objects, to mere things, tools to be used. Men become consumers of the human flesh driven by the sexual instinct as that operating in dogs. The fact that we are made in the image of God to be *anthu* (human) means that all parts of our body participate in this divine purpose as means for the expression of love, care and compassion. There is nothing of this sort between prostituting couples.

The problem of sexual license arises from a misunderstanding of our manhood and womanhood. What does it mean to be a man? What does it mean to be a woman? It has often been said that to be or not to be a man or woman is to be so in bed. It has to do with the mutual sexual satisfaction of men and women. To men this poses a great challenge at various stages in their lives. As a result much of the understanding of manhood is linked with the maintenance of an erection to the point of ejaculation. Viagra has given men a lot of hope, but its side effects are still to be fully known. While this is an important aspect of what men are supposed to be and to do, there is much more to manhood than simply that. It is within this greater view of manhood that we should see male virility. The male "stick" is too vulnerable a part to stake all one's manhood on. Many men know how disappointing the "stick" can be from the way it has often let them down. It is equally unfair, un-loving, and lack of compassionate understanding for women to insist on it since they do not have the same vulnerability. And yet our cultures have invested much in it in their understanding of manhood.

Real men are those who love truly, fully, and deeply with compassion. Love and compassion greatly improve male virility and increase joy because, as the Bible states, "there is no fear in love; but perfect love casts out fear, because fear has to do with punishment. The one who fears is not made perfect in love." (1 John 4:18) Much of the temporary impotence in men and frigidity in women can be traced to all sorts of fears. Real men see themselves as a gift to the other. They lay down their lives for the people they love. It is the love that humanizes them and not the sex.

Real women are also those who know how to love truly, fully, and deeply. Being culturally on the receiving end of men's love, women tend to find loving easier than men and as a result they easily fall victim to unscrupulous men. Most women are constantly in search of men who will love them fully and deeply, but since men often equate love with sex, they do not know how to love fully and deeply. Their love is as ephemeral as their sexual energies. It gets depleted as fast as their sexual tensions. Love is more than sexual tension. When human sexuality is rooted in love, then fidelity comes easily not as a challenge, but rather a delight. What the Apostle Paul advocates in relation to spells of abstinence in order to devote to prayer is regarded as welcome advice in such a loving relationship. Chastity is not only for the celibate state, but also of the married life. The Pontifical Council advises: "In order to live chastely, man and woman need the continuous illumination of the Holy Spirit and that at the centre of the spirituality of marriage lies chastity, not only as a moral virtue (formed by love), but likewise as a virtue connected with the gifts of the Holy Spirit... above all the gift of respect for what comes from God."[32] Extra-marital affairs become unnecessary since they do not add anything to one's manhood or womanhood, let alone to their blessedness. It is satisfactory loving relationships that lead to satisfying sexual relationships. Aiming to promote such relationships will go a long way towards mitigating the spread of HIV/Aids. Both men and women should be taught to acquire their full *uMunthu* and learn how to love truly, fully, and deeply.

The undermining of sexual integrity based on both the traditional and Christian values can be traced back to Independence in 1964. Political freedom was taken to mean freedom from traditional and Christian moral authority. With Independence, Malawi took the path of a secular state in which religion had a role, but a minor one, and moreover, it was not the only moral voice and authority. The MCP became the moral authority in its own right with its Four Corner Stones of Unity, Obedience, Loyalty and Discipline. The churches were relegated to spiritual matters. Teachers were permitted to be polygamous, teenage pregnancies increased, and through the political "*Kabaji ka Banda*" dances popularized by Kanyama Chiume, sexual immorality was considered a human right.

---

[32] Ibid., p. 15.

With the advent of democracy in Malawi, sexual freedom from traditional and Christian norms became one of the new freedoms, and distribution of free condoms due to HIV/Aids seemed to reinforce the freedom. It has been reported by a reputable research organisation that condom distribution has resulted in increased sexual contacts between boys and girls in both primary and secondary schools. This is so because the mere distribution of condoms means society recognises such contact as happening and inevitable, thus giving tacit approval. It is also thought that since they were freely given, they had to be used. This fuels the urge among boys and girls to seek sex when they might not have sought it. Reduced fear of pregnancy and responsibility for pregnancy encourages students especially boys to begin buying condoms. It makes it easy for girls to say, "Yes" and to engage in sex as part of *kunjoya*, to enjoy, and to succumb to the pressure that boys and men exert on them. The result is that sex has become an end in itself, separated from the person who becomes a thing to be used.

This development is not only part of a response to the HIV/Aids crisis, but it is also part of the effects of the global culture. The Sex Revolution that hit America and other Western countries in the 1960's has finally reached us in Malawi. Our people have been exposed to pornographic movies since the liberalization of censorship laws. We are part of the world that has come to believe that sex sells itself and anything else. Beauty pageants are part of it and with the amount of money involved, it attracts many young women. In order to make them morally less offensive, organisers make them look like means of promoting educational and social activities even as female bodies are paraded for public viewing.

It needs to be realised that freedom is responsible since it is a product of love. A state in which anything goes is not freedom, but license. Where there is love, there is truth, and where there is truth, there is freedom, and where there is freedom, there is a deep sense of responsibility for fear of betraying that freedom. Thus, irresponsible sexuality has nothing to do with love and freedom, but has everything to do with licentiousness and moral irresponsibility. It serves the forces of death and not life. Love is life.

To be created in the image of God is to be created in love, with love, through love, by love, and for love. It is to be made a *Munthu* having *uMunthu*. To have *uMunthu* is to have truth, freedom, and responsibility. This means that all human rights and duties are 'love rights'. It is only in having the full right over one's body that one can be a gift to the other. It is only as one possesses full *uMunthu* that one can be a proper gift to another person. To be sexually immoral is to alienate one's sexuality from not only one's person-hood, but one's spirituality as well. It is to lose one's *uMunthu* and to degenerate into a beast with a human face.

9. The Tragedy of Arrested Growth

Puberty is a very significant step in our growth process. All cultures recognise this and celebrate its advent with all sorts of rites of passage. However, the onset of puberty is only a beginning and not the end. The growing process must continue in all areas of life, namely, body, mind, spirit and social relationships. The tragedy is that many people do not go beyond the initial stage of development. They suffer from arrested growth. This means that even their view of sexuality is retarded. It is this mindset fixed on sexual gratification that wreaks havoc in various communities. It remains at the level of 'animality' as guided by instinct and holds on to a form of *uMunthu* without the character to complete it. This is the mindset that makes people who are in their forties and fifties behave like teenagers—the sugar daddies and sugar mummies. They have failed to mature with wisdom and understanding. Such maturity comes with much learning, reflection, and discipline. Such development can be speeded up with proper training especially with an educational philosophy focused on *uMunthu* as the real goal of education.

In his novel, *Youth*, J.M. Coetzee, the 2003 Nobel Prize winner for Literature, he has a nameless male character, who is the main character of the story, that suffers from arrested growth, unable to take charge of his own life responsibly, but always waiting to be fulfilled by someone else especially women. He is delusional about who he is and wants to become, and he is often getting himself into a mess. This is what is said of him at one point in his life, "Once upon a time, when he was still an innocent child, he believed that cleverness was the only yard stick that mattered, that as long as he was clever enough he would attain everything he desired. Going to university put him in his place. The university showed him that he was not clever, not by a long chalk. And now he is faced with real life, where there are not even examinations to fall back on. In real life all that he can do well, it appears, is be miserable. In misery he is still top of the class. There seems to be no limit to the misery he can attract to himself and endure. Misery is his element. He is at home in misery like a fish in water. If misery were to be abolished he would not know what to do with himself." Arrested growth is not cured by even university education, tertiary education only makes it worse because while one gains knowledge, one does not gain wisdom.

Coetzee continues to describe how his main character attempts to justify himself to himself and to others, "Happiness, he tells himself, teaches one nothing. Misery, on the other hand, steels one for the future. Misery is the school for the soul. From the waters of misery one emerges on the far bank purified, strong, ready to take up again the challenges of the life of art." Then listen to this rejoinder on the above philosophic justification. "Yet misery does not feel like a purifying bath. On the contrary, it feels like a pool of dirty water. From each new bout of misery he emerges not brighter and stronger but duller and flabbier."[33]

One has to substitute misery with what is called *"kunjoya"*, that illusive desire for the meaning of life especially through sexual encounters. It is the more one has the better life gets, and yet, like misery, it is like bathing in a dirty pool resulting in suffering. The pursuit of *"kunjoya"* robs people of mature wisdom and keeps them perpetually attached to childish behaviour regardless of age, hence the frequent admonition, *"Abambo a mwana, zimene mukupangazo ndi zibwana."* (Father of our child, your activities are childish.) There are many people, both men and women within society at large and in the church who suffer from arrested growth. Their *uMunthu* is compromised and distorted.

The prevalence of arrested growth is a sign that the Church has failed in its educational endeavours. It has been good at creating members who are half-baked instead of producing disciples as Jesus commanded. Authentic humanness as we find in Jesus is the true target for our growth. His was humanness full of grace and truth and as such it manifested the true glory of the Son of God. It follows then that the more Christ-like we are, the more human we also become. We need to move church members from a membership mode to a discipleship mode in order to bring about behaviour change that is going to help in the struggle against HIV/Aids.

10. Understanding Loneliness, Sexuality and Spirituality

The problem of being alone is affecting many people. There are young people in urban areas out of college and just starting to earn a living who are feeling lonely. There are many young widows with young children to raise, and yet feeling lonely for lack of suitable companions in their lives. There are also old widows who are lonely because they have no grandchildren around them and no male companions as friends due to cultural reasons.

---

[33] J.M. Coetzee, *Youth*, New York: Vintage, 2002, p. 65.

Most of these are in the rural areas. In the past, they would have been inherited, but not any more. While widowers marry younger women within a short time of the death of their wives, older widows are culturally prevented from remarrying at all, if they cannot be inherited. Now even that possibility is being taken away from them due to the threat of HIV/Aids. The situation is bound to increase unfaithfulness, as the number of young widows rises due to the impact of HIV/Aids. Widowed women would wish to have sexual liaisons with men who are more often than not married to other women. They may also wish to have children with these men to fulfil their maternal instincts. Cultural sexual norms notwithstanding, death of a spouse does not automatically commit the widowed to a celibate life. Traditional cultures had their way of dealing with such situations. No young woman was sexually left starving except in observance of certain taboos. They were all remarried. Even the unmarried Makewana had a visiting "python". Is monogamy the only option for legitimate sexual relationships? Is there not a hint that some ordinary Christians were polygamous who were forbidden to take up a leadership role? (1 Tim. 3: 2, 12; Titus 1:6) The implication is that there were people in the church that may have had multiple wives and were being excluded from leadership roles. Even where polygamy is practised, monogamous relationships are regarded as the social norm and are often in the majority. Nevertheless, it is not a case of either/or, but both depending on the circumstances of the particular family and the individual man. The challenge for the Church is to assist such a group to manage their sexuality without the feeling that they are living in sin. The critical question is what is the nature of sexual sins? Is it only men who are involved in sexual sin since they are the only ones who are supposed to lust after women? Why is it that sexual sins are rated higher than other sins? Is monogamous relationship the only legitimate sexual relationship and all others are sinful? How do celibates deal with their sexuality especially those who are religious so that those who are widows and widowers can learn how to manage it without causing scandal? How should people deal with sexual guilt? Does our theology of sexuality and marriage fit the biblical testimony? These are not easy questions, but need to be asked and dealt with.

Here are some of the Biblical statements that are used to speak authoritatively about aspects of our sexuality, but are often used out of their biblical as well as their historical and cultural contexts. "It is not good that a man should be alone" (Gen. 2:18). "It is good for a man not to marry" (1 Cor. 7:1). "Do not deprive each other except by mutual consent and for a time, so that you may devote yourselves to prayer" (1 Cor. 7:5). "For it is better to marry than to burn with passion" (1 Cor. 7:9). How do we reconcile all these positions? How do we relate them to our current situation in the 21st century? There is a lot of selective use of the Bible in its application to moral issues. What can we learn from the actions and attitude of Jesus in dealing with some of the moral issues related to HIV/Aids today? It is said of Jesus that he had compassion on the people. Would that be the key to developing a moral attitude in the context of HIV/Aids?

It seems that it is commendable to be alone for spiritual reasons, and also to be not alone for sexio-spiritual reasons. It is also recommended that sexual relations be suspended for the sake of devotion to prayer. It is the feeling of being alone, which is not a good thing, and that demands that a sexual companion be found. Loneliness is bad, and companionship is good even if it means non-sexual companionship. Spirituality is relational and so is sexuality while being alone is contrary to the human social constitution. Nothing is as terrible as being alone at night and sick. Children or grandchildren may provide needed company, but can never be companions. There is need for a companion who can touch you where very few people would touch you and that with love. The plight of the lonely is a serious pastoral issue. Therefore, we need a strategy that raises these critical questions and a forum to discuss them and come up with relevant theological perspectives.

One of the critical areas to be tackled quickly is that of the use, misuse, and abuse of the Bible. There is need to convene an ecumenical gathering of scholars, preachers and teachers of the Bible to discuss this problem in relation to sexuality. In view of the condemnation of the infected, the discrimination and stigma that accompanies that condemnation, and the effect on the children, the Church needs to initiate this study/consultation quickly. A proper reading and understanding of the Bible, its proper use in preaching, teaching, counselling and pastoral work can contribute much towards eradication of discrimination and stigma. This should be viewed within the context of church outreach, with genuine love (Rom. 12:9ff) to embrace the infected and affected and create space for all those who are vulnerable, in order to encourage them in their faith journey and promote their spiritual growth and renewal.

11. The Condom Debate

In 1999 the Malawi Council of Churches came up with a policy statement on condom use. It stated that while the churches are not in the business of distributing condoms, they recognise that the condom could be used on medical advice. They regretted their failure to teach clearly on matters of sexual morality, but committed themselves to doing so in future especially on abstinence and faithfulness in marriage. This was a major positive response to the issue of condoms. In February 2001 there was a one day State-Faith Communities Consultation at Le Meridien Capital Hotel, which was chaired by the Vice-President, the Right Honourable Justin Malewezi, MP. At that consultation the faith communities agreed with the government on abstinence, and being faithful but disagreed with it on condom distribution as a method in the fight against the spread of HIV/Aids. Their disagreement was largely on moral grounds. While the consultation was a major breakthrough resulting in the formation of the State-Faith Communities Taskforce of which I later became chairperson, the debate on condoms has continued.

Recently Malawi Network of People Living with HIV/Aids (MANET) have challenged the churches to come up with alternatives for fighting the spread of HIV/Aids since they are opposed to the condom. The Advocacy Officer of MANET, Mr George Kampango, is reported to have said, "It is now time to fight the epidemic other than being at each other's neck on petty issues like campaigning against condom use when we know people need them for protection. Let us see the reality on the ground, every day people are dying of Aids, so every one has a role to ensure that lives are saved."[34] This same item was reported in WCC Press News.

Therefore, condom use is what is called a harm-reduction strategy. Professor Tsung-Hsueh Lu of Cheng Kong National University, Taiwan, defines harm-reduction programmes in the following manner.

> "[They] are not intended to cure diseases, nor fully eliminate the risk of diseases, but to mitigate the effects of inherently risky behaviours. Because they assume that some level of risky behaviours will persist, they aim to limit the harms that might befall those who engage in these risky activities. The proponents of harm reduction believe that the behaviours of those involved could not (or are very hard to) be changed, thus we can only reduce the harm."[35]

Of course, the opposite view argues that risky behaviours should not be encouraged, but rather stopped. Therefore, it follows that making condoms available can only encourage unethical behaviour. These two positions can be applied to abortions involving teens and the making available of the

---

[34] Francis Tiyanjah-Phiri, Nation Online, October 7, 2003.
[35] Conference Paper.

morning after pill, to drug use and the supply of syringes, and other situations.

It needs to be admitted here that while the Church has generally condemned condom distribution on moral grounds, it has not clearly spelt out alternatives nor vigorously defended abstinence and faithfulness. It therefore seems that the Church is merely obstructionist in the struggle against the spread of HIV/Aids. It uses the condom debate as a diversionary tactic. It is time the debate was put in its proper context.

From the moment the first case of HIV/Aids was diagnosed in Malawi in 1985, the government was in a state of denial even though we all knew by then from the Ugandan experience with the 'slimming' disease that we were in for a crisis. It was not until almost ten years later that we took the epidemic seriously and started setting up structures for dealing with it. Non-Governmental Organisations, especially Population Services International joined forces with radio messages, posters and condom distribution. The blitz of information on HIV/Aids and condom use disturbed the moral sensitivities of the nation. The approach was quite insensitive to cultural feelings on sexuality and sexual body parts. The Church was also offended for a number of reasons: blunt openness on matters shrouded in secrecy and surrounded by taboos, going against the norm of self-control and wide condom distribution seemed to send the message that sex was acceptable as long as one had a condom for protection. It took away the fear of pregnancy and, therefore, made it easy for as many boys and girls as possible to indulge in sex as long as they had the condom. The sinful aspect of extra- and pre-marital sex was ignored and it became sex on demand. As the condoms were not entirely reliable, it was foolishness to encourage the very activity that had brought about the disease. Therefore, the Church's reaction has been based on a number of concerns. The whole situation is one of confusion as to what is the real problem and how to go about solving it. So, what is the problem?

The real problem is the death dealing impact of HIV/Aids. Returning to Malawi from the USA after an absence of ten years, it was like returning to a war zone. Many friends had died, others were dying and many more have since died. I was General Manager of Christian Literature Association in Malawi and in three years I buried seven members of staff. When I left CLAIM, there were still others who were sick and have since died. There are queues at our mortuaries and our cemeteries are filling fast. The number of orphans is increasing and the social burden on grandparents and relatives is getting heavier by the day. *Mutundu wa aMalawi ukutha* (the nation of

Malawi is being depleted). Even though HIV/Aids spreads through a variety of ways, the main route is sexual intercourse. This is not the only disease that is spread in this manner. There are other sexually transmitted infections (STI), which have never affected the nation in the same way as HIV/Aids has done. The difference with the other diseases is that they have a known cure, and condom use is advised clinically. People die from these other STIs due to carelessness and neglect of their condition. These sexually transmitted infections do not affect the immune system, only certain parts of the body. Therefore, HIV/Aids is in a class of its own.

While the response to the presence of other STIs is personal, private, and a matter of the health service providers, the impact of HIV/Aids has made it a public matter and a concern for everybody. In the past, those infected by what was seen as an epidemic were quarantined to prevent its spread. Most STIs have not been considered as epidemics warranting raising a public outcry. The Government and NGOs have opted for the nation-wide indiscriminate distribution of condoms as the first step in the prevention of the spread of HIV/Aids even though it is presented in documents as the third option after abstinence and being faithful. Therefore, it is against the public face of HIV/Aids and the presentation of the condom as the only effective means of prevention that the Church has reacted rather negatively.

The reaction of the Church was informed by its moral teaching on sexuality, notwithstanding the fact that some church members and leaders are equally guilty of immorality and that some of them have also died of Aids-related causes. To the HIV/Aids crisis, the initial attitudinal response was that people were only reaping what they sowed. It also took the form of a message in a children's song "*Usalire waziyamba wekha*" (Do not cry, you brought it on yourself"). There seemed to be a quiet satisfaction that "We told you so."

The promotion of the condom was like adding spiritual insult to a spiritual injury. It was adding sin upon sin. The condom is not like a bandage that is used to prevent further harm, but something that is going to be used for the same immoral act that brought the disease in the first place.

Furthermore, there was a social dimension to the distribution of the condom that seemed to elude the distributors. Sexual intercourse is physically between two individuals, but in a culture where there are no individuals but corporate persons, sexual intercourse is symbolically between two families. This is the only context in which homosexual language is allowed when male in-laws refer to their brother in-law as "our husband." When condoms are distributed to youth in disregard of their parents' knowledge and counsel, a major social taboo has been breached. This is why condom distribution has been offensive even to the traditional culture. It only helps to further alienate the youth from their culture and their society. This alienation brings more confusion and later, more psychological problems that modern society is not equipped to address. Western NGOs coming from an individualistic culture do not appreciate this social dimension to the free distribution of condoms to school-children. The approach is too individualistic, too mechanistic and too utilitarian.

In order to treat a disease, we do not treat the symptoms unless they are side effects to the disease. By fighting condoms, we are struggling with symptoms of perceived immoral behaviour. The problem is the human heart, spiritual and theological ignorance, inadequate Christian education and failure to love the sinner.

Therefore, for the Church, there are three battles, the medical, the social and the moral one. For the Government and NGOs, it is only the medical problem and the moral one is personal and private. Is the demarcation so clear between the public and the private? Is this not the case of *"Nkhuyu zodya mwana zinapota wankulu?"* ("What the children do affects the elderly.") It also follows that much that is done in private may affect the public domain or what an individual does also affects the community. Is the public domain indifferent to immorality? Who is the public? What is the use of our criminal justice system if it is to remain not moral?

How then do we resolve the impasse between concern for the medical problem and for the moral problem? I do not see any easy resolution here. The real challenge for the Church is to come up with alternatives for the prevention of the spread of the HIV/Aids disease that will be effective and also morally acceptable, since the condom is not. To this challenge the Church has insisted on abstinence or chastity though that is easier said than done. Abstinence relates to pre- and extra-marital relationships. It is a hundred percent foolproof. The risk is zero. The problem is that it is not a hundred percent practiced. The churches know this and most of their discipline cases are about this. So what is the morality that they are defending? The Government and NGOs are reading hypocrisy. The Church is not honest with itself and with the public. There is no Christic realism and praxis.

The Church's other alternative is what the Government and NGOs also acknowledge but know that in many cases it is not working. Couples are generally not faithful to one another. Why should they be faithful if it is a relationship based on *kunyengana*, that is, mutual deception as per the language use? To seduce is not to love as we have established. It is far from it. Love is used as bait and no more. Sexual relationships with anyone and everyone has become an end in itself. Truck drivers and others engaged in trading have become Aids carriers on the various routes that they ply. For many women, poverty has become their undoing.

Why is it that these two approaches have failed? Is it part of Christian idealism, that is, concentrating on what ought to be the case rather than what is the case? Are we not like Peter who said that he was prepared to die for Jesus, but when the moment came, he denied his master? What moral lesson should the Church draw from that for its own moral teaching and guidance of its membership? The Church has failed because it has forgotten the New Testament moral realism and the grace of God.

What other alternative is there for the Church to advocate? I would like to suggest this New Testament moral realism that we see in Jesus, in the apostolic writings, and in the Early Church.

12. Christic Moral Realism and Praxis

Of all human problems, God has identified the problem of the Power of Sin as the fundamental human problem and the source of all other problems. Therefore, it is not surprising that Jesus came into the world to save sinners from this power. Through faith in Jesus Christ, the Power of Sin over individual lives and communities is broken and the power of the life-giving Holy Spirit put in its place for the promotion of a new life of love and justice. The mission of the Church is to proclaim this new life as available to humanity. Jesus did not come to condemn, not even Judas, and so also the Church should not condemn anyone. Jesus fulfilled the role of the Suffering Servant of whom it is said, "A bruised reed he will not break and a smouldering wick he will not snuff out. In faithfulness he will bring forth justice; he will not falter or be discouraged till he establishes justice on the earth. In his law the islands will put their hope." (Is. 42:3,4) This has to be the attitude of the Church to the sinner whether infected or not. This is the love that will never disappoint anyone. Jesus loved the sinner and so must the Church, which should exist for the good of the sinner.

Jesus specializes in searching the lost and rescuing them from danger. The parables of the Lost Sheep and the Lost Coin are about his ministry. There are also many prodigal children who want to come home who need to be welcomed and not rejected. We were all prodigal children at one time. Let us always remember that Jesus came to seek and save that which was lost. (Lk. 19:9)

New Testament Christianity was a religious movement for inclusivity and therefore broke down many walls of separation. It overcame discrimination and stigma against the Gentiles, and against women. It liberated Jews and Gentiles alike. It was a religious movement based on love. At the Council of Jerusalem, Peter said that by giving the Gentiles the Holy Spirit, God showed that he made no distinction between Jews and Gentiles (Acts 15:6-11). Paul declares, "You are all sons of God through faith in Christ Jesus, for all of you who were baptised into Christ have clothed yourselves with Christ. There is neither Jew or Greek, slave or free, male or female, for you are all one in Christ Jesus." (Gal. 3:26-28; see also Eph. 2:11-18)

St. Paul takes up the issue of condemnation and says that no one has a moral right to judge and condemn anyone for it is before one's own master that one stands or falls. To judge is to usurp God's prerogative, that is, to play God. The Church is called to be merciful, as the heavenly Father is merciful. In the discussion on meat offered to idols, St. Paul demonstrates that two opposite actions could be right, that is, abstaining and eating as long as God was being thanked. Could it be that those who are distributing the condom to save some lives from contracting the disease might be equally doing a commendable job as those who are insisting on abstinence? We may actually be fighting a useless battle in God's eyes. The disease has to be fought as well as the moral battle. It is not one battle but two. It is the weapon that we are fighting about.

The moral question has a number of levels on which it can be considered. While the ecclesiastical level is important, it does not provide the bottom line. The bottom line is not the individual conscience, but God's final judgement. Jesus spoke of forgiving seventy times seven times over the same sin or mistake that the offender repents from. The mercy of God is able to cover many sins. For many, falling into sin is not a simple routine, but a real moral struggle that only God knows. *Ambiri a ife kugwa mu uchimo sidala ayi, koma kumpunthwa ndithu.* Remember Rahab the prostitute who was used by God, not only to rescue the spies, but also to become a great great ancestor of our Lord? What about the Samaritan woman and also the woman caught in adultery? There is no sin too big for God's mercy and forgiveness. The Church can be no more scandalized by sin than God is, and if God is able to forgive, what is the Church that it cannot forgive? Morality cannot be legislated, but taught. It cannot be enforced by supervision, but by personal vision. It cannot be maintained by sacramental sanctions, but by opening up the Lord's table to sinners. In the final analysis, morality is between the individual and God. Morality is the life of the Holy Spirit finding expression in our lives for the fruit of the Holy Spirit are: "love, joy, peace, patience, kindness, goodness, faithfulness, gentleness, and self-control. Against such things there is no law. Those who belong to Christ have crucified the sinful nature with its passions and desires." (Gal. 5:22-25) Christian freedom entails liberty from the power of sin and from the law. It also entails liberty for responsible selfhood and for God and not from God.

If the fight against the condom is the wrong battle that is being fought over a weapon for the wrong reasons, what is the right battle that the Church should be fighting and the right weapons to give to people to use? HIV/Aids and condoms are symptoms of a given disease. We do not have to fight the symptoms. Another pandemic is corruption, which has passed crisis levels. Yet another pandemic is incapable and ignorant leadership. The other pandemic is that of women's oppression. The root cause of all these pandemics and problems is the **Power of Sin.** It causes us to live sub-human lives in sub-human cultures of violence, greed, corruption, and oppression. We are going through a deep moral crisis of global proportions and yet modern human civilization continues to be in denial of this lethal power.

It is this moral crisis that the Church should be fighting against. In order to do this, the Church must have faith in Jesus as God's answer to human problems and then present an adequate view of Jesus. The world requires a Jesus who is big enough for its problems and not simply for the soul. We are now reaping the bitter fruits of soul theology that separated the spirit from the body. The Jesus we present is too small and too futuristic to be of any present good. Secondly, the Gospel is still the Good News. We need to discover afresh what is good about it for the present. The early church turned the world upside down, but now the world has turned the Church upside down. We need to recover our natural position and turn the world upside down again. This means developing confidence in our message to transform lives for the better. We are once again to be the salt of the earth and light of the world. However, this can happen when we adopt a discipleship mode from within the Church. Currently we are like salt that has become tasteless and is being trodden under foot because it is of no use to any one.

13. Conclusion

We need to separate the two issues, namely the medical and the moral. To the medical issue, we recommend that the Church says "Yes" to condom use for the prevention of the spread of HIV/Aids as a morally acceptable position and response to the crisis. To be HIV positive is not to cease to be a sexual being. People need to be protected since we are our bothers' and sisters' keepers. On the issue of sexual immorality, the battle is elsewhere, so we are not going to waste time on the condom. It has to do with radical discipleship. We need to engage real causal issues and not symptoms.

Bibliography

Bird, Joseph and Lois, *The Freedom of Sexual Love*, Mumbai: St. Paul Publishers, 2001.
Coetzee, J.M.; *Youth*, New York: Vintage, 2003.
Lai, Hsi: *The Jade Dragon*, Destiny Books, 2002.
Leonard, Bill; *Becoming Christian: Dimensions of Spiritual Formation*, Louisville: Westminster/John Knox, 1990.
Pittenger, Norman, *Making Sexuality Human*, Philadelphia: Pilgrim Press, 1970.
Pontifical Council; *The Truth and Meaning of Human Sexuality*, Nairobi: Paulines Publications, 1997.
Prokes, Sr. Mary Timothy, *Towards a Theology of the Body*, Grand Rapids: Eerdmans, 1996.
Ross, Kenneth (ed.); *Faith at the Frontiers of Knowledge*, Blantyre: CLAIM-Kachere, 1998.
Ross, Kenneth, Following Jesus and Fighting HIV/Aids, Edinburgh: St Andrew Press, 2002.
Thielicke, Helmut; *The Ethics of Sex*, Grand Rapids: Baker, 1964.
Terrien, Samuel, *Till the Heart Sings*, Philadelphia: Fortress Press, 1985.

Related books from the Kachere Series

Dubbey, John, *Tlamelo. The Church Against Aids*, 135 pp.
Fiedler, Klaus, *Let's Build the Bridge*, 20 pp.
Fiedler, Rachel NyaGondwe, *Coming of Age: A Christianized Initiation among Women in Southern Malawi*, 92 pp.
Ham, Frank, *Aids in Africa: how did it ever Happen*, 229 pp.
Kanjo, Chipo, *Will to Live*, 52 pp.
Kholowa, Janet and Klaus Fiedler, *In the Beginning God Created them Equal*, 28 pp.
Nhamo, Kudzai. *A Silent Battle*, 102 pp.
Saur, Maria, Linda Semu and Stella Hauya Ndau, *A Study of Gender-Based Violence Nkhanza in three Districts of Malawi*, 90 pp.
Treasuring the Gift. How to Handle God's Gift of Sex. Sexual Health Learning Activities for Religious Youth Groups, 100 pp.
Fiedler, Rachel NyaGondwe, *Chenjerani, Matenda a Edzi Alikodi*, 24 pp.
Fiedler, Rachel NyaGondwe, *Be Careful. Aids is Real*, 24 pp.

www.ingramcontent.com/pod-product-compliance
Lightning Source LLC
Chambersburg PA
CBHW031555300426
44111CB00006BA/330